# NATURAL HOMEMADE BEAUTY

## 90 Recipes for Skin, Hair and Home

Leoniek Bontje

Photographs by Anya van de Wetering and Bella Thewes
Translated by Kerry Gilchrist

BATSFORD

**Disclaimer**

This book has been compiled with the utmost care. Always exercise caution when you are using plants for medicinal purposes. If you have any symptoms or queries, always consult a doctor. You should also exercise caution with plants if you are pregnant. If you have any uncomfortable physical reactions, stop what you are doing immediately. Neither the author nor the publisher are in any way responsible for problems or injuries caused by using plants.

First published in the United Kingdom in 2024 by B.T. Batsford
43 Great Ormond Street
London WC1N 3HZ

An imprint of B.T. Batsford Holdings Limited

© 2022, Uitgeverij TERRALannoo BV.
For the original edition.
Original title: Plant & cosmetica. Voor huid, haar en huis.
Translated from the Dutch language
www.terralannoo.com

© 2024, B.T. Batsford Ltd. For the English edition.

ISBN 9781849948760

A CIP catalogue record for this book is available from the British Library.

10 9 8 7 6 5 4 3 2 1

Reproduction by Rival Colour Ltd UK
Printed and bound by Toppan Leefung Printing Ltd, China

This book can be ordered direct from the publisher at www.batsfordbooks.com, or try your local bookshop.

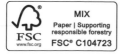

# CONTENTS

# INTRODUCTION

Do you enjoy nourishing your skin with natural products containing wonderfully aromatic plants and flowers? Or how about bathing in flower-scented water and pampering your hair with natural haircare products? It really is the ultimate indulgence, particularly if you can make those products yourself!

Many everyday medicinal plants and flowers are nourishing and replenishing; ideal for looking after your skin. Marigolds and camomile are healing, soothing and calming, while yarrow helps wounds to heal. Oats are nourishing – for your hair too – and restorative for skin suffering from breakouts, rashes and chickenpox.

Your skin is your body's largest organ and its primary function is protection, forming a barrier between you and the outside world to keep out harmful substances. The ingredients in care products that you apply to your skin also enter your bloodstream, so making sure that they are pure, natural and non-toxic is essential.

The average pH of skin is 5. If that value changes, it means that your skin's protective function has been disrupted and it will lose moisture, dry out and become more sensitive to external irritants. You should always try to keep your skin in good condition and avoid applying too many irritating chemicals.

Products that you buy in the shops are often full of ingredients with long, unpronounceable scientific names – and some of them may be harmful to both your skin and the environment. Other ingredients are simply far from natural!

Another issue is that beauty products are often tested on animals; something you might want to avoid when choosing your care products. And, last but not least, good natural skin care tends to be pricey. The solution is to make your own beauty products. You can do this using nourishing medicinal plants growing around you or in locations that are easy for you to access, as well as incorporating natural basic products like olive oil, apple cider vinegar and pure honey from your local beekeeper.

Some people go so far as to say that anything you put on your skin should be pure enough for you to be able to eat it. This applies to things like oil pressed from fruit seeds and vegetables, including carrot oil, broccoli-seed oil, avocado oil, tomato-seed oil and cucumber-seed oil, but you can also use raspberries, sea buckthorn berries, rosehips, coffee and cocoa on your skin.

It doesn't matter how many nourishing products you apply externally; if you want beautiful skin, it is just as important to eat a healthy and balanced diet. You need to take a holistic view of both aspects because your skin reflects how you are feeling and how healthy you are. If I've been eating chocolate or French fries with mayonnaise, then I can tell that my skin looks much worse than when I've been eating fruit, vegetables and grains.

The book that you are holding describes the plants that are good for your skin and gives recipes so you can use them to make your own care products, from marigold ointment to carrot oil. I also share my conversations with various experts along with their recipes. The result is a book that you can use to nourish and nurture yourself, from top to toe.

**Leoniek**

# THE BENEFITS OF MAKING YOUR OWN BEAUTY PRODUCTS

More and more people are researching how to make their own beauty products from plants that they either find growing in the wild or grow themselves. They are turning their backs on all those little pots filled with complicated ingredients that they don't recognize and going back to basics. To making things with pure, simple ingredients.

The main benefit of making your own beauty products is having full control over what you put in them, what type of texture they have and which essential oils you use to make them smell wonderful. Homemade products are also more affordable and the recipes in this book will show you just how easy it is to make your own face, hair and body-care products. Many of them even use products you'll find in your kitchen cupboards and pantry.

Taking responsibility for what you put on your skin feels good; after all, you know what works best, don't you? One of my personal priorities is to choose ingredients that have been grown in an environmentally friendly manner. Many beauty products contain palm oil, for example, which tends to be chemically processed, with the derivatives listed on the packaging.

The oil is then processed further into lots of different chemical ingredients, making it difficult to work out whether a specific beauty product actually contains palm oil. If you choose to make your own beauty products, you can replace palm oil with organic coconut oil.

It's often difficult to establish where aloe vera comes from but I try to find organic options for that as well, and the honey I use comes from a local beekeeper.

Another priority for me is making sure that products haven't been tested on animals and I always use medicinal plants, ideally ones that grow in the wild. And on that note, familiarize yourself with what can legally be picked in the wild and make sure you never pick in abundance or strip out a plant in any one location.

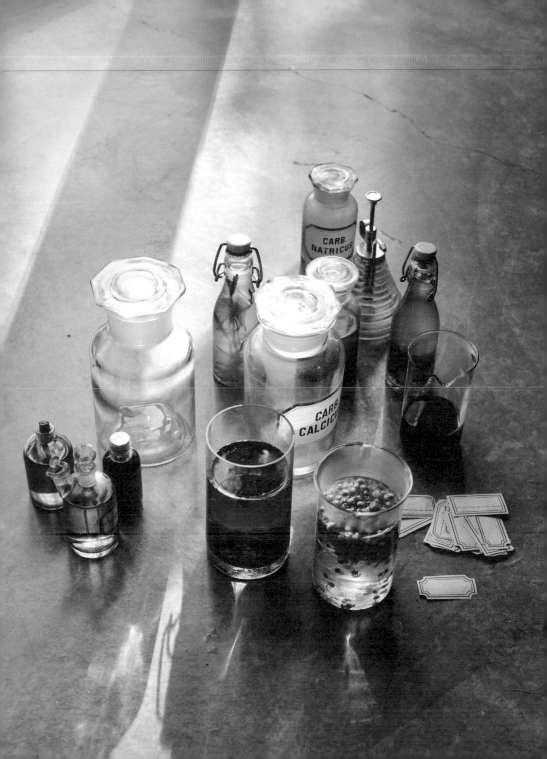

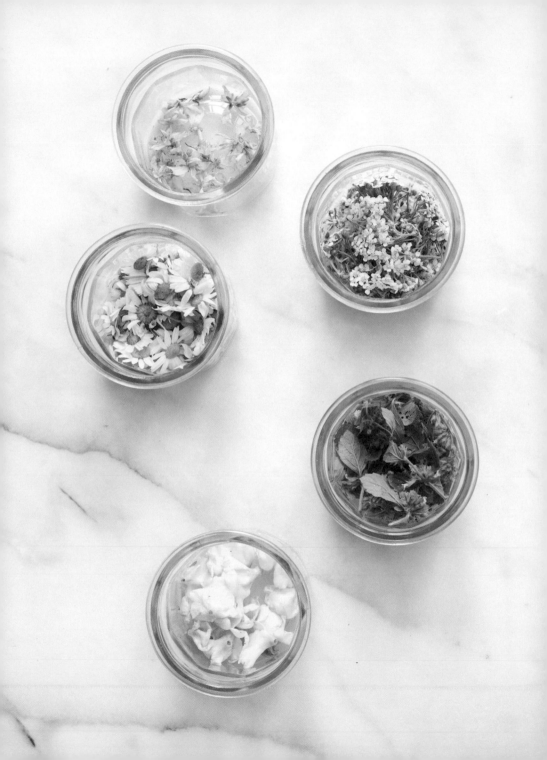

# PLANTS FOR YOUR SKIN

There are lots of plants with healing and/or soothing properties that you can apply directly to your skin:

- Camomile is soothing and you can add the flowers to boiling water for a steam bath, for example.
- Use ground ivy on minor wounds to speed up healing; briefly chew a leaf and then apply as a poultice. You can also rub the leaf on insect bites or nettle stings.
- If you've cut yourself, simply place a leaf from the ribwort plantain on the wound as a kind of dressing. Alternatively, rub it on insect bites or nettle stings.
- Leaves from the dead nettle are another remedy for nettle stings; simply rub them on your skin – they also have soothing properties.
- You can apply yarrow leaves directly to a bloody scrape (if it is bleeding lightly) or rub the juice into pimples and blemishes.
- Marigold has healing and disinfectant properties for minor wounds.
- You can use St John's wort as a kind of iodine and it will soothe sunburn.
- Rose petals have an astringent effect on your skin, so they will help wounds to heal.
- Cucumber slices are perfect for easing tired eyes and cooling sunburnt skin.

- Adding oats or oatmeal to your bathwater will soothe conditions including chickenpox and eczema.

Other plants to use on your skin include heart's ease, sage, witch hazel, common poppy, cornflower, pine, eucalyptus, tea tree, lavender, rosemary, borage, common comfrey, chickweed, catchweed (cleavers), horseradish, arnica, oats, aloe vera, greater celandine and lemon balm. And for your hair, birch, stinging nettle, oats and greater burdock.

## Warning

Although many of the plants in this book are good for your skin and hair, not all plants are harmless. When writing this book, I have assumed that readers are physically healthy, even though I refer to some skin conditions and plants that may help resolve them. If you suffer from severe skin problems, your first port of call should always be a doctor; this book is intended to supplement mainstream healthcare, not to replace it.

Be cautious in the plants you use if you are pregnant or take prescription medicines, or if you are using the products on babies. As a rule of thumb for all plants, stop using something if it doesn't feel good or if you have an allergic reaction.

# GETTING STARTED

How do you get started with making your own beauty products? I begin by choosing a nourishing or healing plant and then exploring what I can make with it – tinctures, oils or ointments – and how I can use it. I think about whether I'll dry the plant or use it to prepare an infusion. You can also begin at the other end and think about what you want to make – a day cream, for example. The next step is to find a suitable plant, like marigold. You can either follow the recipes in this book to the letter and use the plants I specify, or you can decide which plant works best for you and use that one instead. If you want to replace marigold with mallow in your cream, or combine both, then that's completely up to you. Play around with ingredients and create your own personal products.

## Materials

Make sure that all your materials and equipment are clean. If you spend a lot of time making your own beauty products, then keep a separate set of kitchen equipment for this purpose: a hand-held blender, bowl, measuring jug, precision weighing scales, spatulas, stirring rods and so on.

Other helpful tips include collecting all the cosmetic, jam and other pots you can get your hands on, along with their lids (clean them thoroughly by putting them through the dishwasher and boiling them); buying labels or making your own; collecting bits of string and elastic bands; and buying muslin to strain your products. Finally, always label each pot with the product name, ingredients and date.

## Basic ingredients

Your ointments and creams are based on tinctures, infusions, oil macerations and oxymels. These are all prepared using plants so the healing properties of those plants are absorbed into the alcohol, oil, water or vinegar. Read on to find out how to do that. I've used 'plant parts' as a term throughout because you use the leaves and stems of some plants and the flowers or roots of others. The plant descriptions further on in this book tell you which parts of each plant to use.

## Alcohol-based tinctures

You can add a tincture to your ointment or use it to make a compress, and you can also apply it like iodine to a minor wound – a tincture of St John's wort, for example. Take a clean pot and fill it with plant material. Add good-quality vodka, gin or cognac (any spirit with at least 40% alcohol content will suffice) to cover the plant material. Label the pot with the date and contents. Leave for 4–6 weeks with the lid on, shaking occasionally, then strain through muslin. Decant the tincture into a small pipette bottle and it is ready for use.

## Glycerin-based tinctures

If you prefer not to use alcohol, you can replace it with glycerin; a sweet-tasting, plant-based liquid. The method is the same as for alcohol-based tinctures, simply use glycerin instead of alcohol.

Tinctures have a shelf life of approximately two years.

## Macerates and oxymels

You can leave plants to macerate in vinegar, cocoa (made with warm plant milk) or honey to create a simple medicine. If you want something more powerful, prepare an oxymel by macerating the plant parts in vinegar with honey.

**Leaving plants to macerate in apple cider vinegar:** Fill a clean pot with the plant parts and add good-quality apple cider vinegar to cover the material. Leave

to stand for around two weeks, strain and it's ready for use.

**Leaving plants to macerate in honey:** Repeat the above process, adding runny organic honey instead of the vinegar to cover the material. After a few days, the honey will become watery and your oxymel is ready for use.

Oxymels have a shelf life of approximately one year.

## Infusions and decoctions

You can use an infusion on a compress or to rinse your skin or hair.

**Making infusions:** Fill a jug with plant parts, boil water, leave it for a few minutes to cool slightly, then pour over the plant parts in the jug. Leave the infusion for a few more minutes to cool further, then use it to saturate a clean cloth or dressing. Squeeze out excess liquid and place on the skin. Leave for at least ten minutes or overnight to absorb. You can also rinse your hair and skin (or even wounds) by pouring an infusion over them. You can leave some soothing plants to infuse in cold water – for example, mallow, marsh mallow and verbascum. Leave them overnight in cold water, then strain and use the following day.

**Making decoctions:** This involves boiling some plant parts along with the water, such as roots, bark or pine needles. Add two to three teaspoons of plant parts to 500ml of water, bring to the boil and leave to simmer gently with a lid on the pan for approximately 15–20 minutes. Strain to remove the plant parts and leave the decoction to cool before using.

## Macerated oil

Infused – or macerated – oil is made by leaving plant parts in oil to infuse. You can apply macerated oil straight to your skin or use it as the basis for an ointment. You can macerate marigolds in oil, as well as camomile, yarrow and common comfrey – the process is the same for all plants, unless the instructions tell you otherwise.

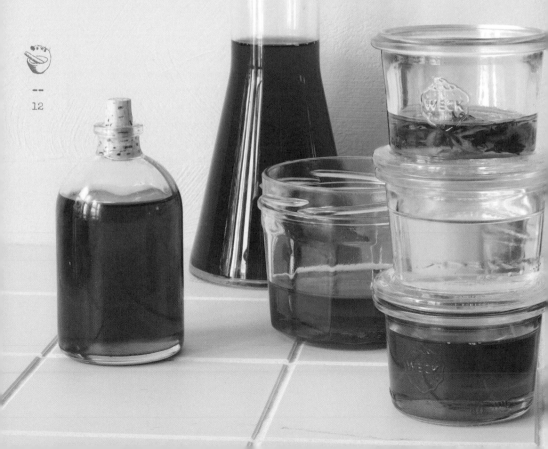

Use almond, sunflower or jojoba oil that is neutral, organic, ideally cold pressed, and not strongly fragranced (see pages 19–21 for a list of oils). You can use fresh plant parts; try to pick them around midday on a dry day, once the dew has dried. Leave them to dry slightly before using. If fresh plant parts are not available, then you can also use dried ones.

There are different ways of macerating plants in oil.

**Cold maceration:** Pick the plant parts, dry them as thoroughly as possible and place in a clean jar (e.g. a jam jar). Pour oil over them to cover the material and mix properly to remove any air bubbles. Stick a label on the jar and cover with muslin and string or an elastic band. Place in a bright location (St John's wort can be placed in direct sunlight). Stir briefly every day with a clean spoon or spatula. After four weeks, strain the oil and either decant into a dark bottle or keep in a dark place.

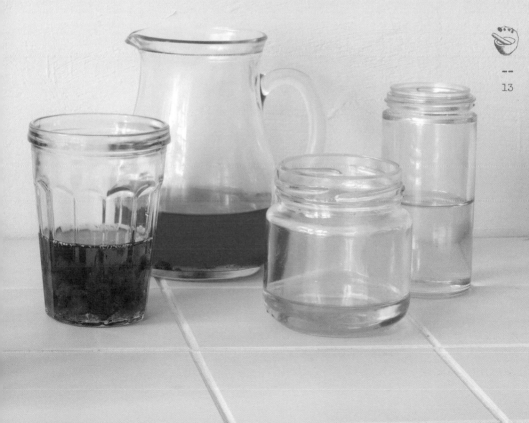

**Warm maceration:** Place the plant parts in a clean jar (e.g. a jam jar) and pour oil over them to cover the material. Place in a water bath and heat for 48 hours, stirring occasionally. A word of caution: don't let the water boil, as that will fry the plant parts. With that in mind, turn the heat off at night and on again the next morning, so you can monitor it consistently. Stir regularly. After 48 hours, strain the oil through muslin or a fine sieve and decant into a dark bottle.

Macerated oils have a shelf life of approximately six months to one year (or as long as they smell good).

## Ointment
## (oil- or fat-based)

### Ingredients for approximately 250ml

- 200ml infused oil (see pages 12-13 for macerated oil recipe) or 100ml coconut oil and 100ml vegetable oil
- 20g beeswax
- The more beeswax you use, the thicker the final product will be. For lip balm, use 40g beeswax for every 200ml oil (1:5). For a smoother ointment, use 10 or 20g beeswax for every 200ml
- (1:20 or 1:10 respectively).
- 20 drops essential oil of your choice
- 10 drops vitamin E oil
- A clean 250ml pot or jar with lid

Melt the beeswax in a water bath. Once the beeswax is fully melted (and not before), add the infused oil and mix (if you heat the beeswax and the oil together, the mixture may catch fire). Then add the essential oil and vitamin E oil, mixing thoroughly. Decant into the pot and leave to set. Then put the lid on the pot and add a label.

Ointments have a shelf life of approximately two years (or as long as they smell good).

## Cream
## (oil- or water-based)

### Ingredients for approximately 250ml

- 70ml organic oil of your choice
- 20g emulsifier such as glycerol monostearate (to make sure that the water and oil mix)
- 170ml distilled water or an infusion of heart's ease, daisy or any other plant of your choice (see page 31)
- 20 drops essential oil of your choice
- 10 drops hydrolate of your choice
- 10 drops vitamin E oil
- A clean 250ml pot or jar with lid

Heat the organic oil in a water bath. Add the emulsifier and stir carefully until it has blended thoroughly with the oil. Bring the water to the boil, then add to the warm oil. Stir carefully until you have a thoroughly blended, smooth mixture – this will probably take several minutes. Then add the essential oil, hydrolate and vitamin E oil. Stir carefully until blended, then decant the cream into the pot.

Make sure that both the pot and your equipment are completely clean as the cream is prone to mould. You could also add a preservative.

Creams have a shelf life of approximately six months.

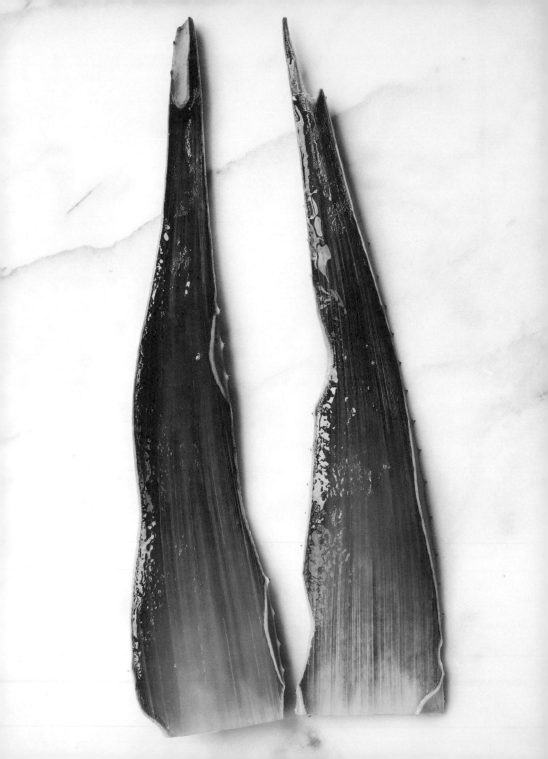

# ALOE VERA
(Aloe)

Asphodelaceae

We use the gel from the leaves of the aloe vera plant as first aid for burns and abrasions to the skin. It is also the ideal water component for creams.

## Effect on the skin
Soothing, softening and hydrating. Boosts healing of wounds, is anti-inflammatory, analgesic and antiseptic, and it improves circulation.

## When to use
On skin that is dry and chapped, first and second-degree burns, sunburn, abrasions, ulcers, acne, cold sores, shingles, fungal infections, age spots, hair and skin that is in poor condition, dry scalp, premature skin aging and stretch marks.

## Active ingredients in the gel
Water, polysaccharides, sterols, enzymes, amino acids, tannins, urea, salicylic acid and vitamins B, C and E. In addition, minerals including calcium, iron, zinc, potassium, sodium, manganese, magnesium, copper, selenium, sulphur, phosphorus, zinc, strontium, cobalt, chromium and tin.

## Use
The gel from the leaf of the plant.

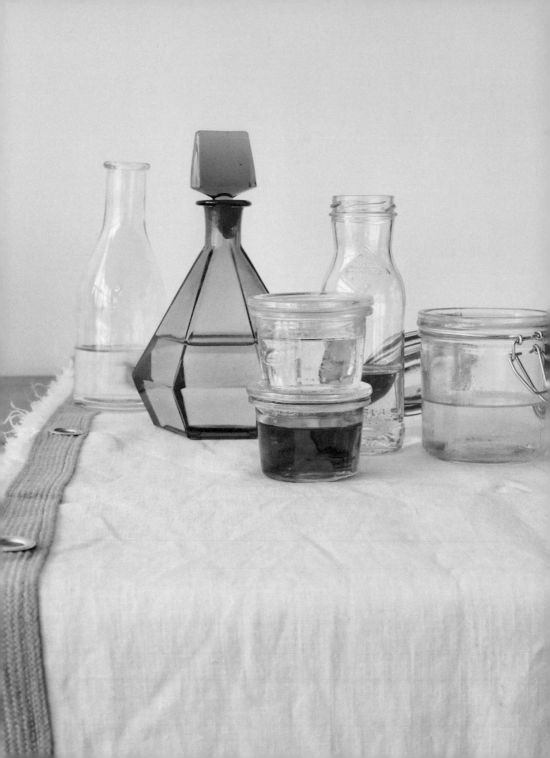

# NATURAL BASIC INGREDIENTS

## CARRIER OIL

There are lots of different types of oil that are safe and beneficial for the skin, so you can use them as the base for your skin- and hair-care products. Try to find a cold-pressed, organic version. This is a list of oils that are commonly used.

### Apricot-kernel oil
Apricot-kernel oil is produced by pressing the kernels from apricots (*Prunus armeniaca*). As the oil resembles the fats that are naturally present in your skin, it is easily absorbed. This oil contains vitamins C and E, along with the unsaturated fatty acids omega 6 and 9 to soften and strengthen your skin.

### Almond oil
Almond oil is a mild oil that is produced by pressing the fruits (almonds) of the almond tree (*Prunus dulcis*). It contains antioxidants and vitamins A, D and E. Particularly suitable for dry, sensitive skin, but it can be used on all skin types. It will combat premature skin aging and promote skin elasticity. The almonds are ground before being pressed for the oil, which is then filtered and bleached.

### Argan oil
Argan oil is extracted from the kernel of the fruits growing on the Moroccan argan tree (*Argania spinosa*). The oil nourishes, hydrates and protects your skin, and it also contains antioxidants to combat premature skin aging. You can also apply it to your hair for a lustrous shine.

### Avocado oil
Avocado oil is extracted from the flesh of avocados, which are the fruits of the avocado tree (*Persea americana*). The oil is used in beauty products as it is rich in unsaturated fatty acids, which are both hydrating and nourishing.

### Borage oil
Borage oil is pressed from the seeds of the herb borage (*Borago officinalis*). It is high in gamma linolenic acid (an essential omega fatty acid) and has many other

excellent properties for your skin, including nourishing it, boosting its elasticity and moisture content, stimulating the production of sebum and encouraging it to repair itself. It combats the symptoms of eczema, acne and psoriasis, replenishes dry skin, reduces wrinkles, combats premature skin aging and strengthens brittle nails and hair.

## Olive oil

The olive tree (*Olea europaea subsp. sylvestris*) bears fruits that can be pressed to make olive oil. Use a light, organic olive oil for optimal absorption through the skin.

## Prickly pear oil

Prickly pear oil is a precious oil that is extracted from the black seeds of the prickly pear cactus (*Opuntia ficus-indica*). Rich in unsaturated fatty acids, vitamin E and minerals, it nourishes, hydrates and strengthens your skin, improves its texture and protects against premature skin aging.

## Castor oil

Castor oil is extracted from the seeds of the green fruits of the castor bean plant (*Ricinus communis*). It is packed with omega 9 fatty acids that nourish your hair, follicles and scalp, stimulating the growth of hair, beards, eyelashes and eyebrows.

## Sea buckthorn oil

The sea buckthorn oil, available commercially, is pressed from the berries and seeds of the sea buckthorn (*Hippophae rhamnoides*), but you can also make your own oil by macerating sea buckthorn berries in oil (see pages 12–13). Sea buckthorn oil contains vitamin A and stimulates cell renewal in your skin.

## Grape-seed oil

Grape-seed oil is pressed from the seeds of grapes grown on grape vines (*Vitis vinifera*). Choose cold-pressed oil whenever you can, so that you get as many nutrients as possible from this strengthening and deeply nourishing oil, which is ideal for sensitive skin.

## Jojoba oil

Jojoba oil is a liquid wax that is extracted from the seeds of the jojoba bush (*Simmondsia chinensis*). It is yellow when pressed but is often bleached before being sold. Jojoba oil is very similar to sebum produced by your glands, so it is hugely beneficial for your skin, cleansing it and preventing it from producing excess sebum. Your hair will also love it.

## Coconut oil

Coconut oil is pressed or extracted from copra, which is the dried, white flesh of the coconut, the fruit of the coconut palm (*Cocos nucifera*). The oil melts at 24–26°C and is liquid in hot temperatures, but tends to set in cooler climates. Coconut oil is a common ingredient in beauty products as it is packed with vitamins and minerals and nourishes, cleanses and disinfects your skin. Make sure that you buy good-quality coconut oil, ideally from a small-scale grower.

## Linseed/flax oil

Linseed oil is cold pressed from the seed (linseed) of the flax plant (*Linum usitatissimum*) and contains omega 3 and 6 fatty acids, along with other unsaturated fats. The oil prevents your skin from drying out and combats premature aging – effects that are enhanced when used in combination with evening primrose and/or borage oil. Linseed mixed with water produces a gelatinous paste that reduces inflammation and draws splinters from your skin.

## Moringa oil

Moringa oil is extracted from the seeds of the *Moringa oleifera*; a tree that is known for its healing properties and high levels of nutrients and antioxidants. The oil is rich in vitamins A, B and C and contains minerals including iron, magnesium and zinc. It sets at temperatures below 20°C and is both anti-aging and hydrating.

## Neem oil

Neem oil is extracted from the seeds of the olive-shaped fruits of the Asian neem tree (*Azadirachta indica*) as well as the fruits themselves. Neem oil is used in Asia as a medicinal oil to repel insects, counter skin infections (such as eczema) and reduce inflammation. The viscous oil is either golden, brown or reddish and has a strong, not particularly pleasant smell. It is also used as hair oil and an ingredient in shampoo.

## Rosehip oil

Rosehip oil is extracted from the seeds of rosehips from the dog rose (*Rosa canina*) and other rose varieties. This deeply nourishing oil contains vitamin A, among other ingredients, and helps to reduce scarring, minimize stretch marks and combat premature skin aging.

## Evening primrose oil

Evening primrose oil is pressed from the seeds of the evening primrose (*Oenothera biennis*) and is rich in unsaturated fatty acids. The oil's high content of gamma-linolenic acid means it helps to reduce inflammation.

## Walnut oil

Walnut oil is cold pressed from the fruit of the walnut tree (*Juglans regia*) and is soothing, healing and slightly astringent. The oil reduces inflammation, benefits dry and more mature skin, and gives some protection against the sun.

# WAXES AND FATS

## Beeswax

Beeswax is extremely hydrating, contains vitamin A and will not block your pores, so it is an ideal base for creams. It is also anti-inflammatory and antibacterial, so it is effective against breakouts and blackheads, plus it nourishes your scalp and hair follicles. Beeswax melts at between 62 and 65°C, but it starts to soften at 40°C, so holding it in your hand will start the process. Beeswax comes from the honeycombs in beehives. Although removing it may seem harsh, a beekeeper friend of mine told me that the honeycombs need to be cleaned annually anyway, which involves removing some of the wax. Try to buy your beeswax from a reputable, reliable beekeeper or producer. Beeswax is an animal product so it is not vegan.

## Candelilla wax

Candelilla wax is a good plant-based alternative to beeswax. It is extracted from the leaves and stems of the candelilla bush (*Euphorbia antisyphilitica* or *Euphorbia cerifera*) that grows in desert areas in northern Mexico and the southwestern United States. Boiling the leaves and stems releases the wax, which is then processed further to clean it. Candelilla wax melts at 70°C, so it is slightly harder than beeswax. It can be used to thicken creams and is ideal for chapped skin and sensitive baby skin.

## Carnauba wax

Carnauba wax is extracted from the leaves of the carnauba palm (*Copernicia prunifera*) that is native to Brazil. Beating the leaves releases the wax, which is then refined and bleached. Carnauba wax is harder than both candelilla wax and beeswax and melts at 85°C.

## Shea butter

Shea butter is a common ingredient in beauty products. It is derived from the nuts of the African shea tree (*Vitellaria paradoxa*), which are dried and then processed into shea butter. Shea butter melts at 27°C, contains vitamins A and E and is used in ointments, lotions, soaps and hydrating creams.

## Cocoa butter

Cocoa butter is extracted from the seed of the cacao tree (*Theobroma cacao*). The cacao beans are ground into a kind of fatty pulp – the cocoa mass – which is pressed to separate out raw cocoa butter and cocoa powder. The cocoa butter is sometimes refined to remove its colour. Cocoa butter melts at around 36°C (so it is classified as butter).

## Wool fat

Wool fat (also called lanolin) is derived from sheep's wool and can sometimes be used as a base for creams. Wool fat is ideal for treating extremely dry and cracked skin. It smells of sheep – which attracts some people and puts others off. Wool fat melts at 42°C.

## Vaseline

This jelly-like product can be used as a base for creams. As it is a byproduct of petroleum, I prefer not to use it for skin care products. Vaselines melts at between 40 and 60°C.

# ESSENTIAL OILS

Pure essential oils are derived from plants, flowers and resins, although synthetic equivalents are also available. I asked Frank Bloem, perfume maker at The Sniffaroo, about the differences (see also pages 216-219, where Frank explains how fragranced candles are made).

Frank: 'Essential oils are highly concentrated fragranced oils that are present in some plants. They have different purposes, including protecting the plant against damage or attracting insects. Essential oils are often a blend of fragrances, with the plant itself acting as perfume maker. Essential oils can be extracted from the plant through distillation.' 'Some fragrances have synthetic equivalents. Perfume makers prefer to work with simple (i.e. unblended) fragrances to create

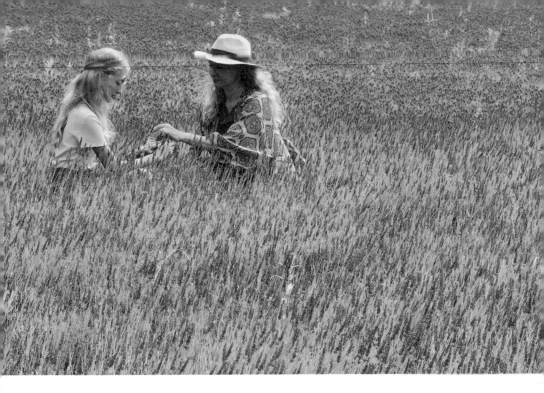

new ones. Some are still extracted from plants, like eugenol (clove oil), while others are reproduced using chemicals.' 'Aromatic oils or nature identical oils are synthetic products; they recreate the fragrance of jasmine, for example, or lavender. From a chemical perspective, the composition is the same as the natural product, but using synthetic ingredients.'

**TIP**
See page 57 for an overview of calming and stimulating essential oils.

Never apply essential oils directly to skin; always mix them with a carrier oil – jojoba or olive oil, for example – by adding 3 to 5 drops of essential oil to 1 to 2 tablespoons of carrier oil.

# LAVENDER

(Lavandula angustifolia)

Lamiaceae

Although essential lavender oil is often chosen for its wonderful fragrance and calming effect on the nerves, this oil is also great for your skin.

## Effect on the skin

Antibacterial, antiviral, antifungal and promotes wound healing. It is also calming, relaxing and balancing and promotes good sleep.

## When to use

On burns and wounds, as well as skin breakouts. It also helps with anxiety, stress and sleep issues.

## Active ingredients

Essential oil, tannins, bitter substances, triterpenes, phenolic acids and flavonoids.

## Use

The flowers or the essential oil.

# PINE

(Scots Pine)

Pinaceae

The first thing you notice about pine is its wonderful resinous fragrance. Both the resin and the essential oil are antiseptic, antibacterial and antifungal, so pine is a natural antibiotic. Pine also purifies the air and helps you breathe properly (this also applies to spruce).

## Effect

Air purifying, cleansing.

## Active ingredients

Resin and gum, essential oil, bitter substances and vitamin C.

## Use

Clippings, needles and essential oil.

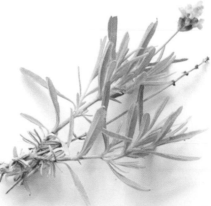

# EUCALYPTUS

(Eucalyptus globulus)

Myrtaceae

Eucalyptus has disinfectant properties and protects against infection. The leaves contain an essential oil that helps you breathe properly, so eucalyptus is a common ingredient in vapour rubs to treat colds.

## Effect on the skin
Antibacterial and antiviral, as well as air purifying.

## Active ingredients
Essential oil – including cineole (also known as eucalyptol) – tannins, flavonoids, phenolic acids and triterpenes.

## Use
The adult leaves and essential oil.

# TEA TREE

(Melaleuca alternifolia)

Myrtaceae

The tea tree was originally only found in Australia but is now grown elsewhere as well. The essential oil is something we all turn to as a matter of course, with many of us using it for its antibacterial, antiviral and antiparasitic properties.

## Effect on the skin
Cleansing. Kills bacteria, fungi and viruses.

## Active ingredients
Essential oil and oxides.

## Use
The essential oil. Mix with a carrier oil (such as jojoba or olive oil).

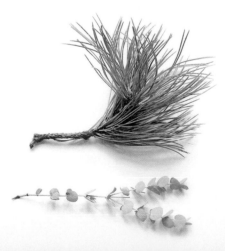

# FRANKINCENSE RESIN

Resinous frankincense crystals come from the frankincense tree, also known as the Boswellia (*Boswellia serrata*, *Boswellia carteri*, *Boswellia frereana* and *Boswellia sacra*). Michelle Dinger from The Ohm Collection imports the pure frankincense resin and explains how it can be used.

Michelle: 'Frankincense oil and lumps of resin are great for helping skin to heal. The resin was originally used to embalm corpses and cleanse holy spaces. These days, frankincense mixed with oil and water is used internally for detoxification. It is both antibacterial and antiseptic. The resin is also often used in skin-care products because it boosts cell renewal.'

Frankincense is also effective against arthritis, inflammation, skin breakouts and acne. Resin from Oman is best, says Michelle. The red kind is very rare, while the white and green resin are easier to come by and of good quality. They are available as balsam, frankincense, crystals and oil.

You could also make yourself a tincture of frankincense and other resins, such as pine resin. For external use, choose 90% (denatured) alcohol. If you want to swallow frankincense (some people do so to boost their immune system), then either add a small piece to hot water, chew on it, or make a tincture with 40% alcohol.

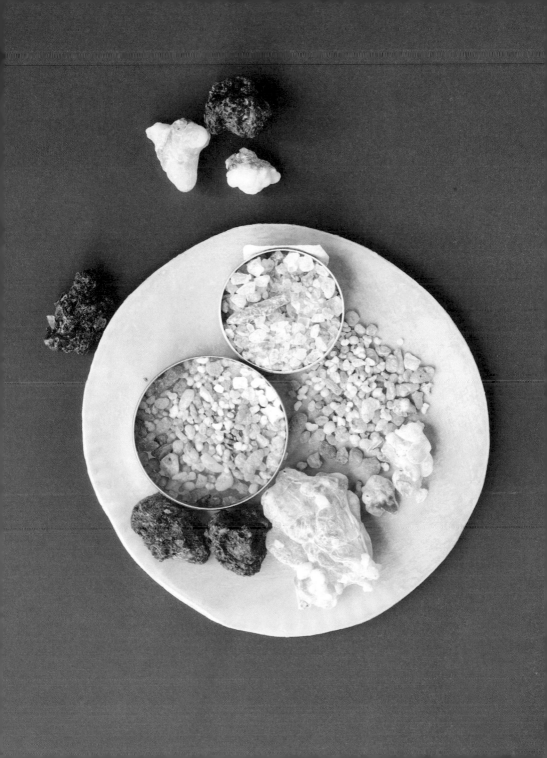

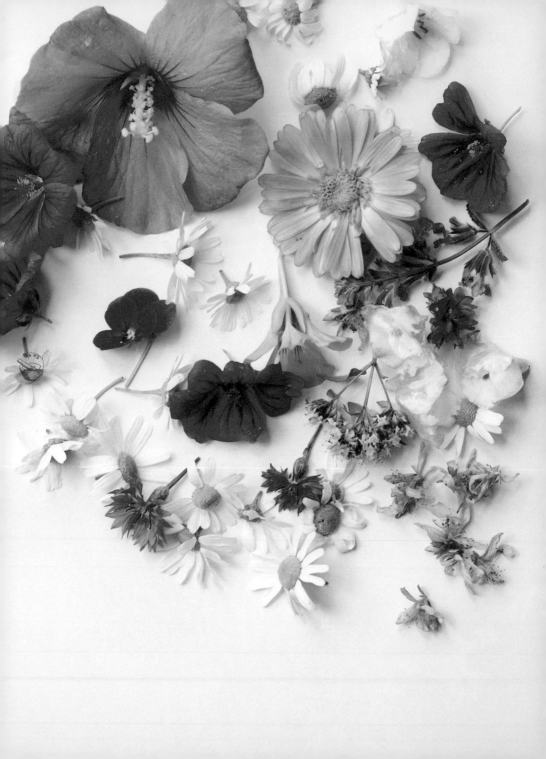

# HYDROLATES

Hydrolates (also known as hydrosols or flower waters) are a byproduct of producing essential oils and a common ingredient in skin-care products. Distillation is used to extract essential oils and hydrolates from plants and the process creates steam containing the soluble plant components. Once the steam is cooled and captured, the floating layer of essential oil is removed with a pipette. The hydrolate is what is left behind. Hydrolates that benefit our skin include rose, lavender, orange blossom, witch hazel, mint, eucalyptus and strawflower (*Helichrysum*).

## Making your own hydrolate

Making your own hydrolate is straightforward, although the notes of the fragrance may occasionally vary. Add water to a pan (don't overfill) and place a steamer basket on top of the pan. Put an empty, heat-resistant dish in the centre of the steamer basket, surrounded by the plant parts. Cover the pan with a domed lid, with the domed side facing downwards. Fill the lid with ice cubes and place the pan on the heat. As the water in the pan evaporates, the rising steam passes around and through the plant parts. Once it reaches the cold lid, it condenses and the droplets trickle around the dome of the lid, before dripping into the dish.

## Hydrolate of the curry plant or bamboo

One very special hydrolate is that of the curry plant (*Helichrysum italicum*), also known as 'immortelle' or 'strawflower'. As well as relaxing, boosting and regenerating your skin, it stimulates your skin's ability to repair itself and is ideal for more mature skin. This hydrolate is also a quick first-aid spray for bruises, contusions and minor wounds, as it reduces swelling and soothes on application. Curry plant hydrolate has a warm, aromatic fragrance. Another wonderful hydrolate is that of bamboo; a grass that is rich in silicon and is stimulating, soothing and anti-inflammatory. Bamboo stimulates the production of collagen and is an excellent tonic for your skin and hair.

# OTHER BASIC
# INGREDIENTS

## Cider vinegar (apple cider vinegar)

You can use cider vinegar to make facial toners and hair rinses. Cider vinegar is a natural, cloudy, unprocessed and unfiltered product that is made from fermented apples. The floating bits that turn alcohol into vinegar are called the 'mother' and they are what lock all the beneficial nutrients into the liquid.

## Baking soda

Baking soda is a common ingredient in deodorants as well as an alternative to shampoo and toothpaste. Use no more than once a week as shampoo. Baking soda neutralizes acids in your mouth, helps to remove plaque, and acts as a light abrasive to polish away any grey deposits on your teeth. To prevent your tooth enamel from being worn away, using no more than once a fortnight as toothpaste.

## Arrowroot powder

Arrowroot powder is a starch made from the roots of the arrowroot plant (*Maranta arundinacea*), which grows in the rainforest. The roots are washed and then ground into pulp. This pulp is then sieved to produce a starch that is dried in the sun. Arrowroot powder is a natural thickener that is used in beauty products and nourishes and nurtures your skin.

## Glycerin

Glycerin is a colourless and odourless liquid extracted from plants. It retains moisture and resembles a natural substance that is present in the top layer of your skin, the stratum corneum. Glycerin is easily absorbed by your skin and it helps in keeping it hydrated.

## Cornflour or cornmeal

Cornflour is made with corn and is sometimes used to bind products, or as a filler – as in deodorants.

## Salicin and salicylic acid

Salicin is found in willow bark and meadowsweet and is metabolized in the body into salicylic acid. The active ingredient in aspirin is synthetic acetylsalicylic acid and some people apply a solution of this painkiller in water to their skin to treat spots and breakouts. Alternatively, you can also use willow bark and meadowsweet for the same purpose. Salicin is a good treatment for acne, inflammation and skin irritation. It also dissolves sebum in skin pores, so it is effective against blackheads and styes. Use primarily on oily, combination and irritated skin.

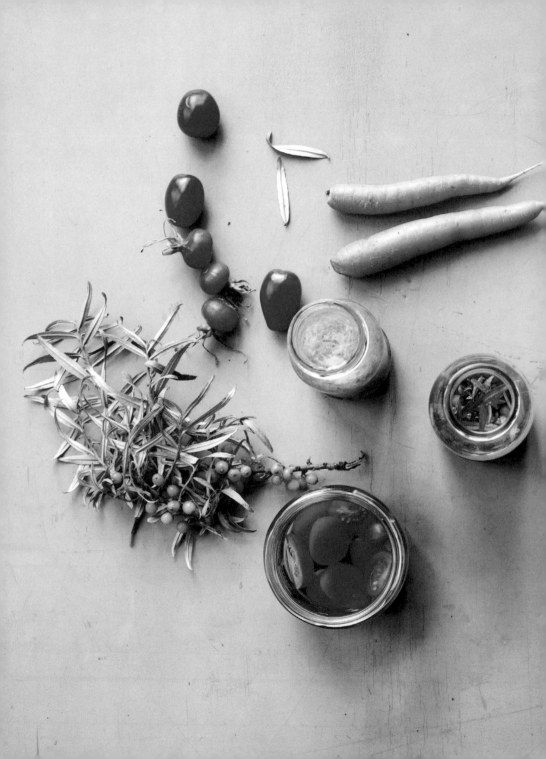

# USING FOOD AS BEAUTY PRODUCTS

More and more people are saying that you should be able to eat whatever you put on your skin and you can also use food to nourish your hair and skin. Some of the kitchen staples that can be used in this way are old favourites — putting cucumber on puffy eyes and sunburnt skin, for example, or using lemon juice to lighten your hair — you can also use the flesh from plums or apricots as a face mask or apply linseed to your skin. Or how about using rice water to condition, nourish and strengthen your hair?

**Carrots** contain vitamin A, which helps your skin to repair itself and stops it from aging so quickly. Use carrots to make a mask or macerate them in oil (see pages 12–13 for details about maceration).

**Broccoli seed** contains vitamins A, C and E and protects against skin-aging free radicals. You can soak the seeds in oil or buy oil pressed from the seeds.

**Sugar** has a restorative effect on your skin and some hospitals apply sugar to patients' pressure sores to help the skin heal. Sugar can also be used as an exfoliating scrub.

**Honey** also has a healing and restorative effect on your skin. Try to use organic honey, ideally from a local beekeeper.

**Coffee** has an antioxidant effect on your skin. You can macerate coffee beans in oil and use coffee grounds as a scrub.

**Oatmeal** has a healing effect on your skin. You can use oatmeal for chickenpox, irritated skin and breakouts, including eczema. Put some oatmeal in a face cloth, tie it together and drop into the bath.

**Cucumber** is cooling, so slice it and apply to puffy eyes or sunburnt skin. Cucumber seed is anti-inflammatory and packed with minerals. You can macerate the seed in oil.

**Rice water** is good for nourishing your hair. Save the water you cook your rice in, leave it to cool and apply evenly.

**Linseed gel** is an excellent styling product, especially on curly hair. Soak linseed overnight in water and use the resulting paste as styling gel or a nourishing mask (see page 136).

**Tomato-seed oil** contains lycopene; an antioxidant that protects your skin against premature aging.

**Pumpkin seed** contains vitamins and minerals and is restorative for your skin.

**Avocado** is rich in unsaturated fatty acids and is both nourishing and healing. Mash the flesh of half an avocado, apply to your skin as a mask and leave for 20 minutes. Avocado oil is both healing and hydrating.

**Banana** is rich in vitamin E and has a hydrating effect. For dry skin, add a teaspoon of honey to a mashed banana. For blemished skin, add a teaspoon of baking powder and half a teaspoon of turmeric powder.

**Raspberries** have an antioxidant effect on your skin, as do sea buckthorn and rosehips. Use them to make masks.

**Turmeric** has anti-inflammatory properties. Make sure you mix it with several other ingredients, as it will dye your skin yellow if you use it on its own.

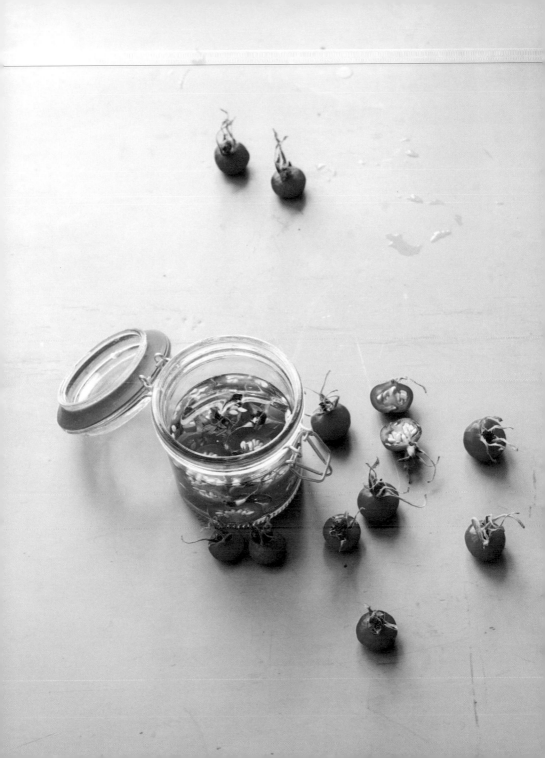

# LOOKING AFTER YOUR FACE

Using home-made products that are tailored to your skin type is a wonderful way to look after your face. If your skin is oily, for example, use aloe vera, lemon, nettle or apple cider vinegar. Oil made from camomile and marigold is a better option for dry skin. The sky is the limit, from a day cream with sea buckthorn, vitamin C and other antioxidants to nourish and protect your skin to a night cream with calming lavender. Or what about a scrub made with rosehip seeds, a steam bath with camomile, a face tonic with yarrow or a face mask made with rosehips and aloe vera?

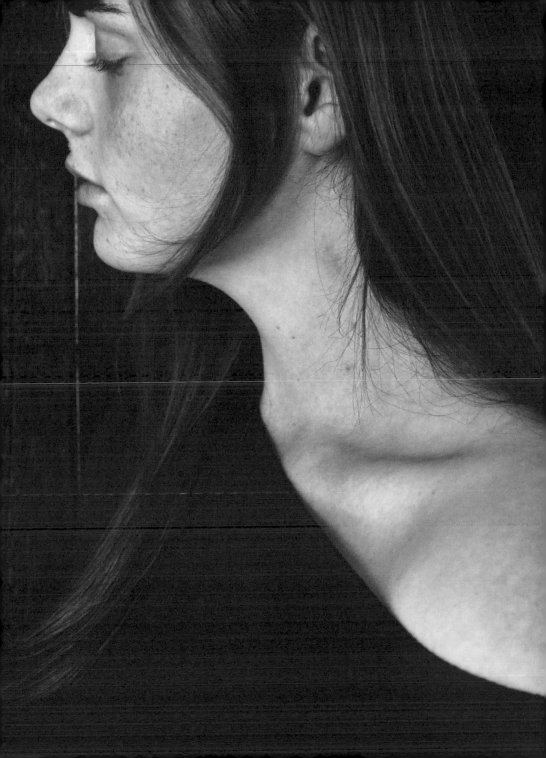

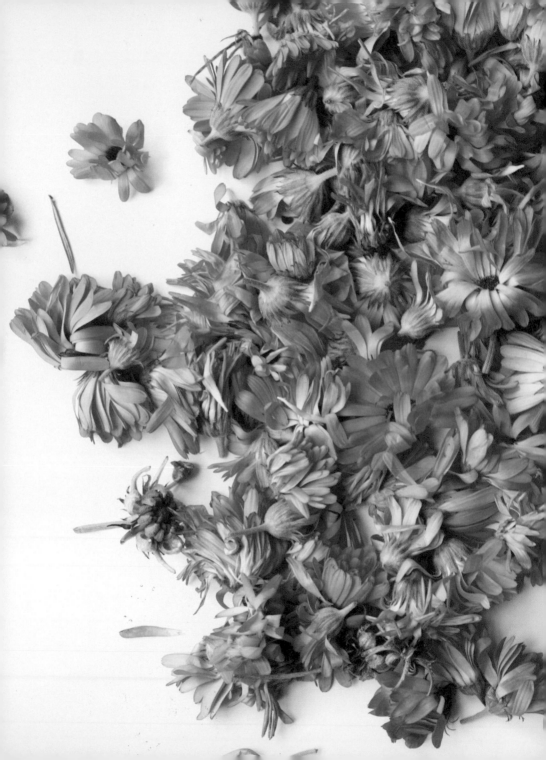

# MARIGOLD
(Calendula officinalis)

Asteraceae

Marigold has beautiful orange/yellow flowers that are good for your skin in many ways, making them an ideal ingredient for your home-made skincare products.

## Effect on the skin
Astringent, soothing, helps wounds to heal and encourages blood clotting. Disinfectant, antibacterial, antiviral and antifungal. Stimulates the formation of new small blood vessels. Marigold contains skin-repairing and healing substances including xanthophyll, allantoin and resin.

## When to use
On cuts, abrasions and superficial wounds. On serious and poorly healing wounds, pressure sores, inflamed skin, hives, acne, boils, eczema, abscesses, piles, dry skin and psoriasis. On cold sores, shingles, fungal skin infections (such as athlete's foot), warts, corns, verrucas, calluses and fissures (nipples and anus). Use marigold oil on nappy rash and bedsores, as well as to encourage skin healing after radiation treatment.

## Active ingredients
Flavonol glycosides, xanthophyll, allantoin, resin, essential oil, bitter substances, calenduline, mucilage, saponins, vitamins A and C, calcium, silicon, sulphur and salicin.

## Use
The flowers. Use only the orange petals for the oil and ointment. To treat wounds, place a leaf over the wound or apply the tincture as iodine. You can also prepare an infusion to apply with a compress.

# MARIGOLD OINTMENT

Start by preparing the marigold oil (calendula oil) that you need to make the ointment.

**Ingredients for approximately 200ml oil**
- 50–100g fresh marigold flowers (enough to fill the pot)
- 175ml good-quality sunflower, olive or almond oil
- A clean 200ml pot or jar with lid
- Muslin

Fill the pot with marigold flowers and add oil to cover them completely. Cover with muslin and leave in a sunny spot for four weeks, stirring daily. Then strain the oil. Or use the warm method with fresh or dried flowers: place the flowers in a bowl and add oil to cover them. Place the bowl in a water bath and warm for approximately 48 hours. Then strain the oil.

**Ingredients for 140ml ointment**
- 20g beeswax
- 120ml marigold oil
- Three 50ml pots with lids, such as cleaned ointment pots

Heat the beeswax in a water bath. Once the beeswax is completely melted, add the marigold oil and mix thoroughly. Pour into the pots, tapping them gently or stirring until any air bubbles have disappeared. Top up to the lip of the pots and leave to set. Put the lids on the pots and apply a label to each one.

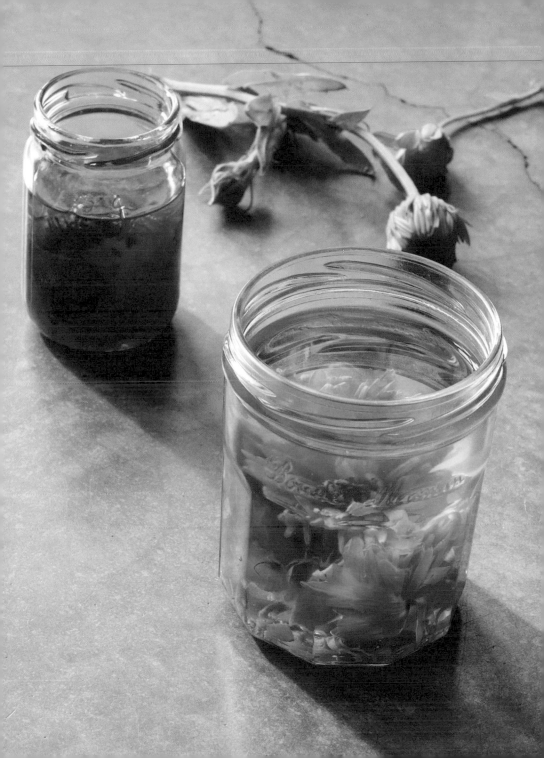

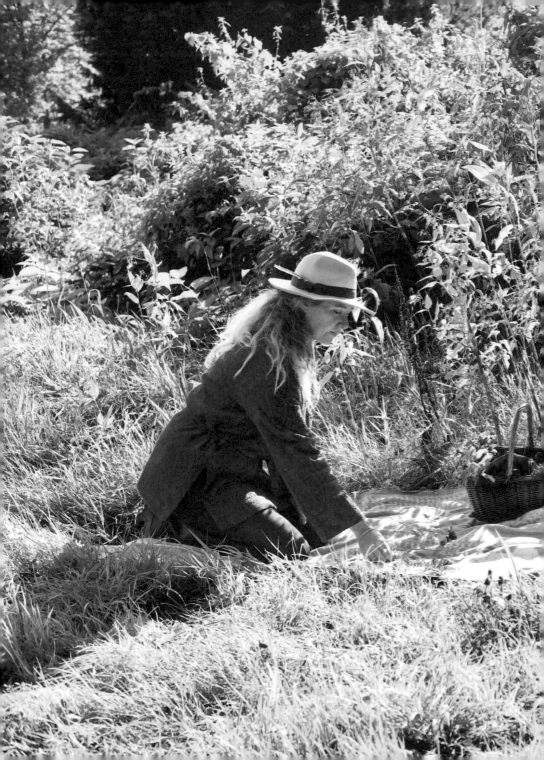

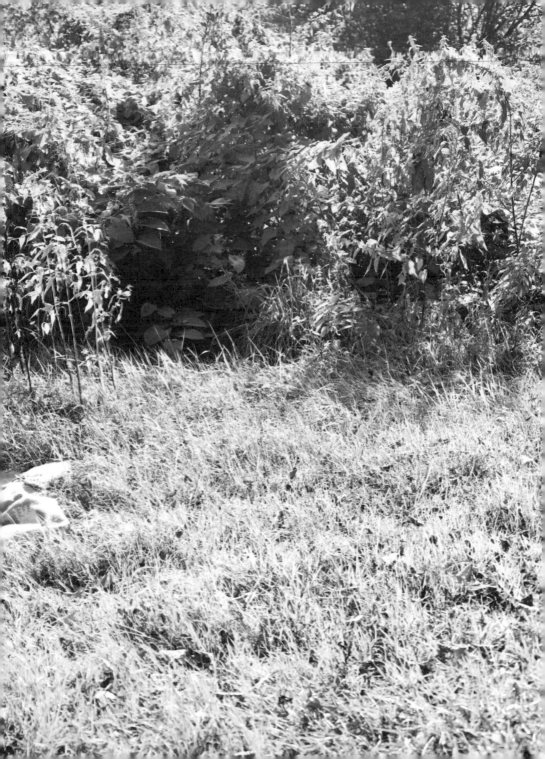

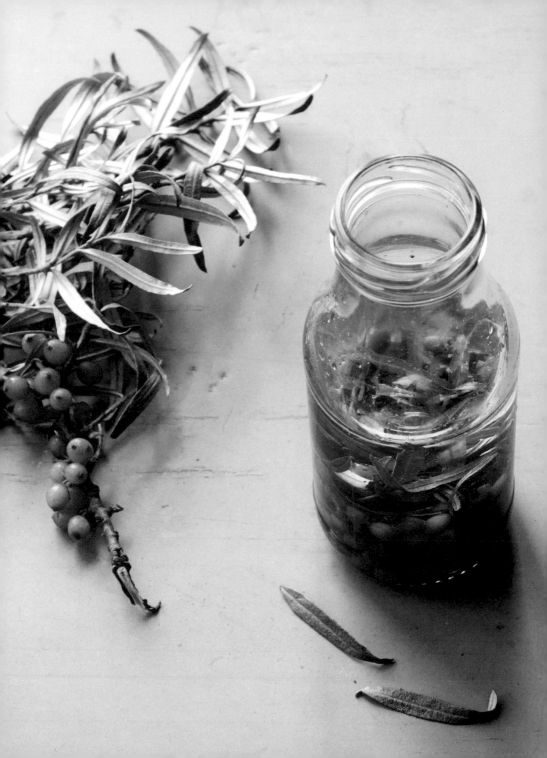

# SEA BUCKTHORN
(Hippophae rhamnoides)

Elaeagnaceae

Sea buckthorn bushes grow on or along the dunes beside the sea and produce my favourite berries. They are rich in vitamin C and wonderful for your skin. Start by using the berries to make oil, then use that to prepare a delightful ointment that is packed with vitamin C and other antioxidants.

The oil that is extracted by pressing the seeds is rich in omega 7 fatty acids that accelerate the ability of the cells in your skin and mucous membranes to repair themselves. The best way to harvest sea buckthorn is to break off twigs carrying the berries (the twigs will soon grow back again) and keep them in the freezer. Strip off the berries before using them.

## SEA BUCKTHORN OIL AND ROSEHIP OIL

Sea buckthorn berries and rosehips are rich in vitamin C and other antioxidants, so they are ideal for nourishing and nurturing your skin.

### Ingredients for 150ml
- 50g (approximately 10) rosehips or two handfuls of sea buckthorn berries (or 50g of a mixture of rosehips and sea buckthorn berries)
- 120ml almond oil or another oil of your choice
- A clean 150ml pot or jar with lid
- Muslin

Cut the rosehips in half and crush the sea buckthorn berries slightly (if you are using them). Fill the pot with the rosehips and/or sea buckthorn berries and pour oil over them. Cover the pot with muslin and leave for four weeks, stirring occasionally. Strain through muslin and the oil is then ready for use.

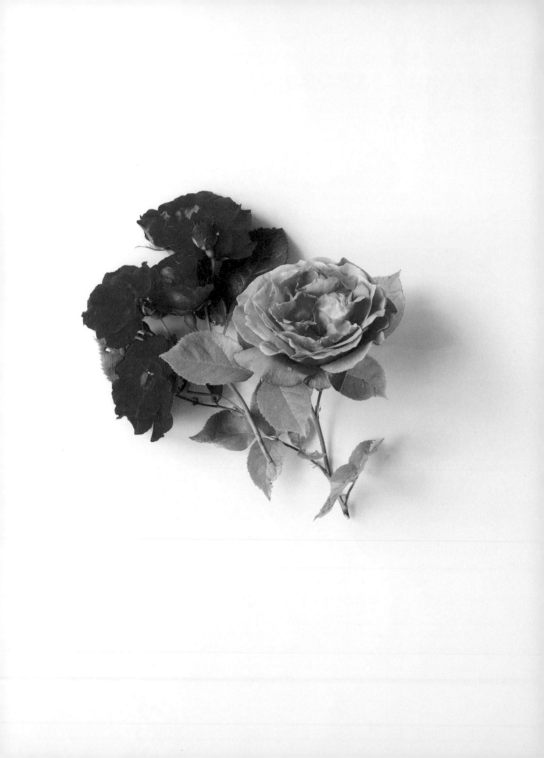

# ROSE
## (Rosa canina)

Rosaceae

This rose is also known as dog rose, wild rose and witches' briar. You can use the rosehips from wild rose bushes in your garden as well as the ones growing wild in hedgerows. They are rich in vitamin C and you can use them to make an effective face mask.

## Effect on the skin
Antioxidant, anti-inflammatory and cleansing.

## Active ingredients
In the rosehips: vitamin C, flavonoids (including rutin), glycosides, fruit acids, tannins, anthocyanins, carbohydrates, pectin, carotenoids and vitamins B1, B2, B3, B5, K and E.

In the seeds: unsaturated fatty acids, essential oils, vitamins A and E, anthocyanins, vanillin and very small amounts of vitamin C.

## Use
Fresh rosehips.
You can dry the seeds to use as a scrub (grind them finely first with a pestle and mortar).
Rose petals are also a common ingredient in beauty products. The fragrance is heavenly and the petals are astringent, encourage blood clotting and help wounds to heal, so they minimize the appearance of your pores.

Use rose petals to make your own rosewater (see overleaf).

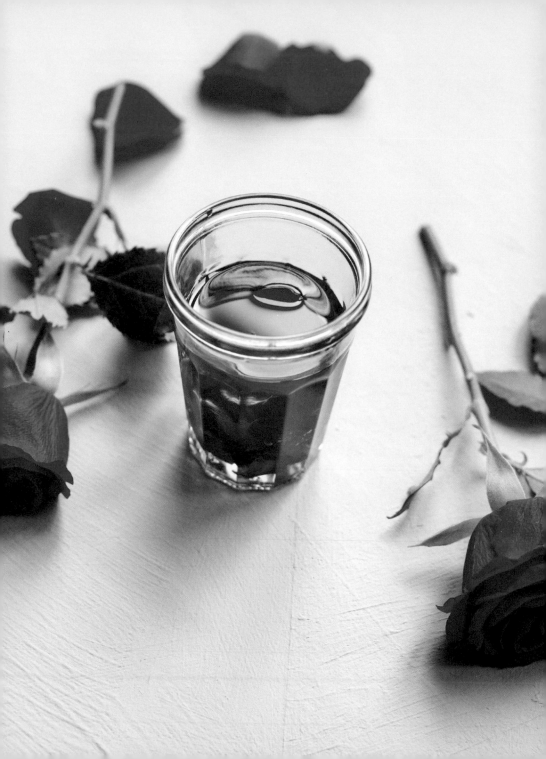

# ROSEWATER

A wonderful daily treatment for your skin.

## Ingredients for approximately 250ml
- 50–100g fresh or dried rose petals (make sure that they have a strong fragrance)
- 300ml water
- A clean 250ml bottle with cap

Put the rose petals in a pan with the water. Bring to the boil and leave to simmer gently over a low heat for approximately one hour. Remove from the heat and leave overnight to infuse. Strain to remove the rose petals and pour the rosewater into the bottle.

See page 31 for instructions on how to make a hydrolate.

# ROSEWATER WITH WITCH HAZEL

This water is a wonderful way to cleanse and nourish your skin.

## Ingredients for approximately 100ml
- 100ml rosewater (see the recipe on the left)
- 15 drops of witch hazel hydrolate (order online or make your own)
- A clean 100ml bottle with cap

Pour the rosewater into the bottle and add the witch hazel hydrolate.

# WITCH HAZEL
(Hamamelis virginiana)

Hamamelidaceae

Witch hazel improves your circulation, including in your skin, so it is a common ingredient in skin-care products. The proanthocyanidins in witch hazel help prevent and reduce cold sores.

## Effect on the skin
Disinfectant and helps wounds heal. Improves circulation.

## When to use
For eczema, itching, rosacea, insect bites and cold sores. Cold sores are caused by the herpes simplex virus; treat with witch hazel hydrolate or a diluted tincture of 1:3 parts water.

## Active ingredients
Tannins, saponins, choline, flavonol glycosides, resin and proanthocyanidins.

## Use
Leaves and bark.
Make a tincture, infusion, hydrolate or witch hazel water (leave the leaves and bark to macerate in water).

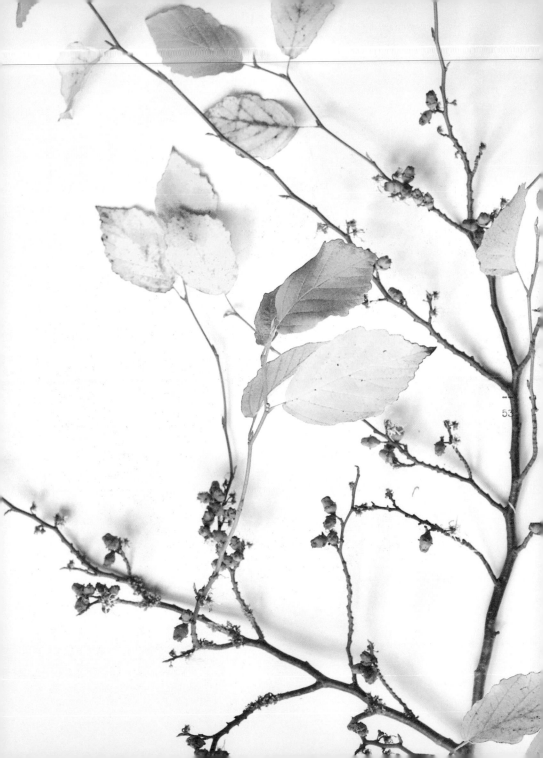

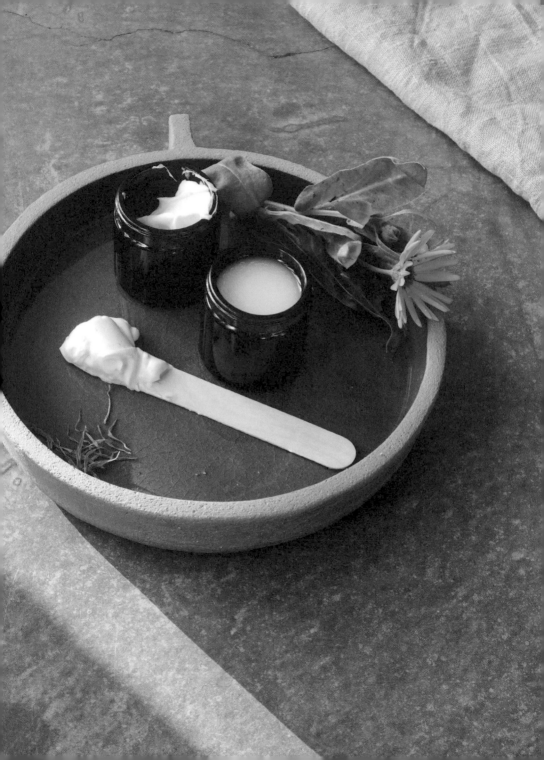

# NELE ODEUR'S DAY AND NIGHT CREAM

Nele Odeur is a wonderful friend and colleague who is dedicated and passionate about the workshops she runs. She is the person behind Scent & Spice, a knowledge and experience centre focused on ethnobotany (how people use plants), where she hosts courses and workshops on plants for medicine, cooking and beauty products. She is also guest lecturer in ethnobotany at Wageningen University. She has narrowed her focus over time to plant constituents, processing plants and how plants affect the human brain.

Nele describes herself as a plant freak, life artist, dream catcher and serial wordsmith. Her interest in how the brain works led her to explore the concept of creativity and how we can incorporate it into how we think and live, and ultimately to create a mentoring programme for creative life artists and dream catchers. Her book about plants, creativity and extraordinary life choices was published in 2022 and is rooted in her passion for telling stories.

Keep reading for Nele's recipe for a day or night cream.

Nele: 'A cream is a blend of water and a fat component. As water and fat don't combine naturally, we also add an emulsifier to overcome that and create a smooth, homogeneous cream.

'We use macerated oils for the fat component; oils that are infused with the active ingredients of plants. See pages 12–13 to find out how to create macerated oils. Check the composition of the fatty acids to see which oils suit which skin types and always choose the right one for your skin. Almond and avocado oil is ideal for dry or sensitive skin, while grape seed and jojoba oil is a better option for greasy or blemished skin. Choose apricot-kernel and jojoba oil if you have normal skin.

'Your options for the water component are hydrolates (distilled plant water), infusions (herbal teas) and decoctions (boiled plant extractions). I prefer hydrolates because the distillation process sterilizes them, minimizing the risk of them spoiling or becoming mouldy. Effective hydrolates for your skin include lavender, orange blossom, witch hazel, wild camomile, rose, elderflower and yarrow – either buy them or make your own. Aloe vera is another ingredient that you can use for your water component.

'Emulsifiers that are commonly used in natural beauty products include glycerol monostearate and cetyl alcohol. Blending the two produces a rich, stable cream that hardly ever goes wrong and is therefore ideal for beginners.

'Because creams contain water, there is a high risk of it spoiling (becoming mouldy). Unless you only make small quantities that you will use within a week or two, I recommend adding a preservative, ideally a natural one.

'Apart from emulsifiers and preservatives, there is a huge range of ingredients that you can add to creams for an extra medicinal or cosmetic effect. These include special ingredients (such as proteins and minerals), nourishing oils (like sea buckthorn and prickly pear oil) and essential oils, which will

also add fragrance. Always wait until the cream has cooled before adding essential oils, to prevent the aromatic substances from evaporating. There are no limits to the potential combinations and added ingredients.

'The only difference between a day and a night cream is the oils and essential oils that you use. Night creams tend to contain oils that are richer and have a higher fat content, so that they can be absorbed into the skin overnight. Using the same oils for a day cream might make your skin feel greasy and leave a shiny layer. Another decisive factor is the essential oils you choose, because essential oils affect the nervous system and the result can range from invigorating through to relaxing. Adding an invigorating essential oil to a night cream could result in disrupted sleep, so always think about how your choice of essential oil will affect your nervous system, not just what it smells like. See opposite for a list of essential oils that can be used in skin care products and how they affect the nervous system.'

**Invigorating essential oils**

Basil
Lemon
Cinnamon
Eucalyptus
Ginger
Grapefruit
Juniper berry
Oregano
Patchouli
Pepper
Peppermint
Rosemary
Sage
Scots pine
Silver fir
Tea tree
Thyme

**Relaxing essential oils**

Benzoin
Bergamot
Cedarwood
Clary sage
Geranium
Jasmin
Lavender
Lemon balm
Mandarin orange
Orange blossom
Petitgrain
Rose
Sandalwood
Vetiver
Wild camomile
Ylang ylang

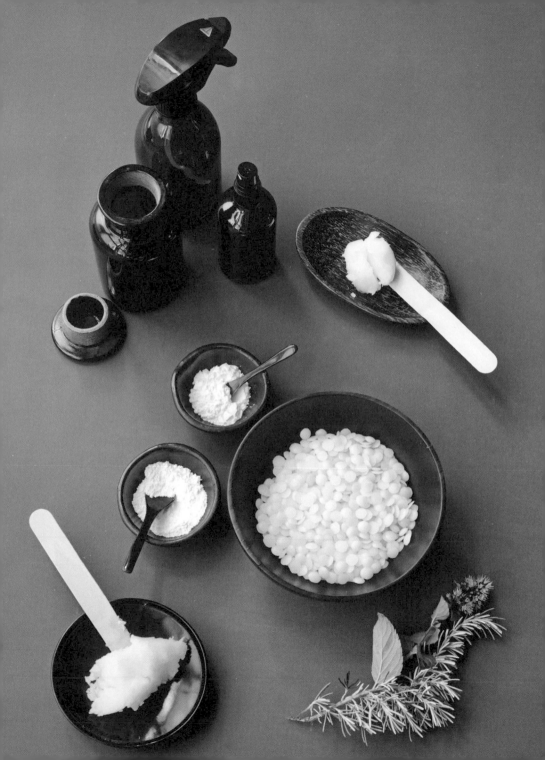

**Ingredients for 100ml cream**

- 20g macerated yarrow oil
- 20g macerated camomile oil
- 10g glycerol monostearate (emulsifier)
- 2g cetyl alcohol (emulsifier and stabilizer)
- 40g hydrolate of your choice
- 20g aloe vera gel
- Optional: 1g rokonsal™ (natural preservative)
- Optional: 20-40 drops essential oil of your choice
- Two measuring jugs
- Thermometer
- Blender
- A clean 100ml pot or jar with lid

Follow the instructions on pages 12-13 or the recipe on page 63 to make macerated yarrow and camomile oils. Weigh out 20g of each macerated oil and put them in the same measuring jug, along with the glycerol monostearate and cetyl alcohol. Put the hydrolate and the aloe vera gel in the other measuring jug. Place both measuring jugs in the water bath and heat to between 60 and 70°C. Once all fats and emulsifiers have melted and both substances have reached the same temperature, remove the measuring jugs from the water bath. Do not skip this step as it is crucial to prevent the cream

from separating. Place the fats in a blender (or use a handheld blender) and mix continuously as you add the water component until a smooth cream forms. This will take a minute or two. Leave the cream to cool to room temperature and add the preservative and essential oil, if you are using them. Put the cream in a spotlessly clean pot and add either a sticky or tie-on label.

**TIP**

You can tweak the proportions when you make the cream. If you want a richer cream, then add more of the fat component – maybe another 10g. Increase the water component slightly if you want a lighter cream.

**Help!**

Sometimes the cream will separate as you make it. It looks like there are little fat pieces floating in the liquid and you can't get them to mix. There are various reasons for a cream to separate, including if the room temperature is too high or the fat and water components are at different temperatures, but all is not lost. Turn the blender to maximum speed and mix as hard as you can. If that doesn't work, try adding a dash of cold water or hydrolate and keep mixing. In 99% of cases, you will still end up with a rich and homogenous cream.

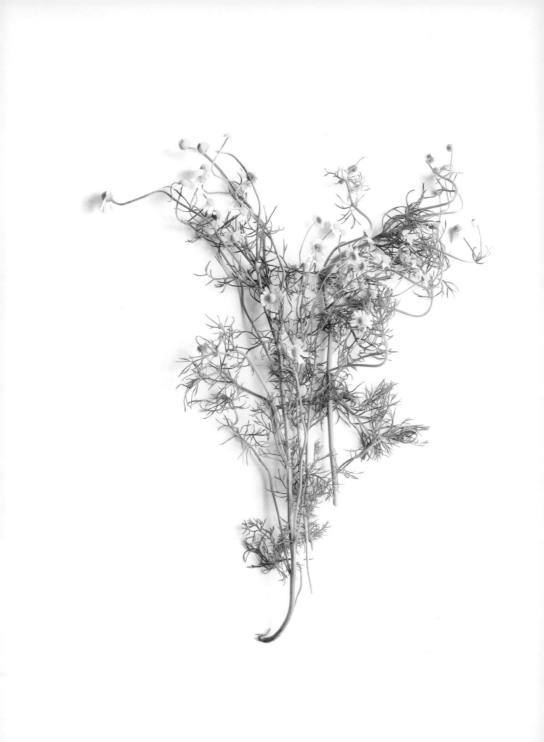

# CAMOMILE
## (Matricaria chamomilla)

Asteraceae

Camomile has wonderful white and yellow flowers that
have a healing effect on your skin and hair, as well as
feathery leaves. You can be certain that you have genuine,
good-quality camomile if the flower head is hollow on
the inside. The plant should always smell strongly of
camomile, so pay close attention to the fragrance.
Applying camomile infusion to your hair in the long-term
makes it wonderfully glossy and will lighten it slightly.

## Effect on the skin
Anti-inflammatory and disinfectant.

## When to use
On poorly healing wounds, pressure sores, eczema and
inflamed skin.
Used together with marigold, it is good for sensitive skin.
It is most effective against fungal infections when
combined with tea tree oil.

## Active ingredients
Chamazulene essential oil, bitter substances, tannins,
mucilage, methyl salicylate, coumarins, flavonoids,
minerals including calcium, phosphorus and sulphur, and
vitamin C as well as choline.

## Use
The flowers for a tincture, tea, infusion or oil. You can
then use the oil as a base for ointments.

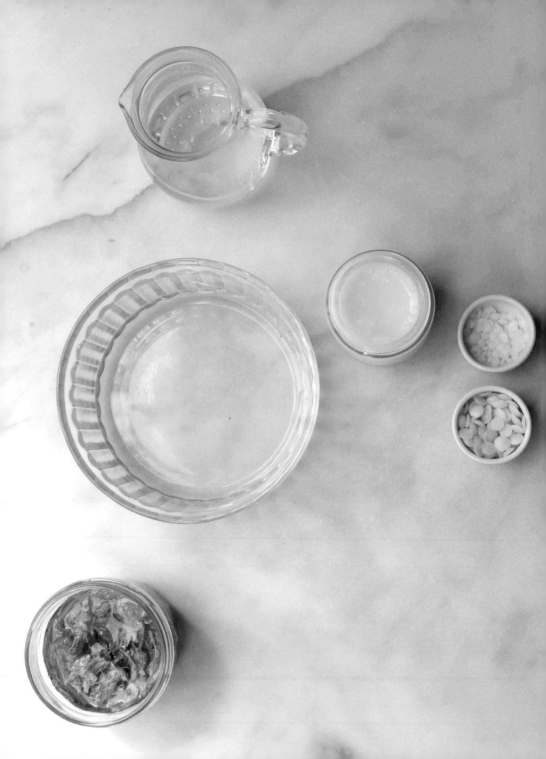

# SOOTHING, COOLING CREAM

This cream is wonderful if you suffer with irritated skin.

### Ingredients for 250ml
- 40ml yarrow oil
- 10g beeswax
- 20g emulsifier, such as glycerol monostearate
- 50ml camomile tincture
- 100ml camomile infusion
- 50ml aloe vera gel (from a tube or squeezed from a freshly picked leaf)
- Optional: 20 drops essential oil, 5 drops vitamin E oil and 1 tbsp witch hazel hydrolate
- Optional: preservative (not required but will extend the cream's shelf life)
- A clean 250ml pot or jar with lid

**The first step is to make the camomile tincture, yarrow oil and camomile infusion.**

**Camomile tincture.** Place 50-100g camomile flowers in a pot, pour over 150ml good-quality vodka and leave for six weeks, shaking the pot occasionally. Strain and the camomile tincture is ready for use.

**Yarrow oil.** Fill a clean pot with 50-100g yarrow flowers and leaves. Pour over 150ml good-quality oil, then cover with muslin and an elastic band. Leave to stand for around two weeks, stirring briefly every other day. Strain through muslin or a fine sieve and the yarrow oil is ready for use.

**Camomile infusion.** Fill a clean pot with 100g camomile flowers – either fresh or dried. Pour over 500ml hot, freshly boiled water and leave to stand for approximately ten minutes. Strain and the camomile infusion is ready for use.

### Then make the cream
Place the yarrow oil, beeswax and emulsifier in a water bath and heat. Place the camomile tincture, camomile infusion and aloe vera gel in a different small pan and heat. Make sure that both mixtures are at approximately the same temperature. Slowly add the camomile infusion mixture to the oil mixture and stir thoroughly until you have a smooth, homogeneous cream. Add the essential oil, vitamin E oil and witch hazel hydrolate (if you are using them), as well as the preservative (also optional). Transfer to the pots, put the lids on the pots and apply a label to each one.

# YARROW
(Achillea millefolium)

Asteraceae

Yarrow's branching stems look a little bit like our vascular system and that is one area that the plant is good for, since it encourages blood to clot and wounds to heal. That makes yarrow an essential part of your first-aid kit for treating abrasions, whether bleeding or not, such as you might suffer in a fall. The Latin name *Achillea* comes from Achilles; the mythical general who used yarrow to treat his armies' wounds.

## Effect on the skin
Stimulates circulation, encourages blood clotting and helps wounds to heal.

## When to use
On bloody abrasions, acne and other skin imperfections.

## Active ingredients
Essential oil, flavonoids, alkaloids, phenolic acids, tannins, coumarins, minerals including potassium, sodium, calcium and phosphorus, and vitamins C, B1, B2 and choline.

## Use
Flowers and leaves. Start by making a tincture (see page 67) and then a blood-clotting and wound-healing spray with one third tincture and two thirds spring water in an atomizer.
Use the flowers and leaves for an oil. Apply directly to your skin or use it as a base for ointments.

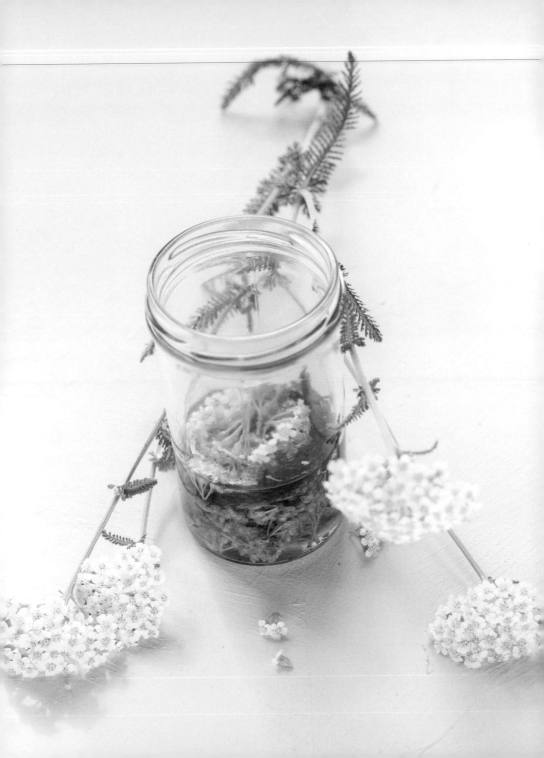

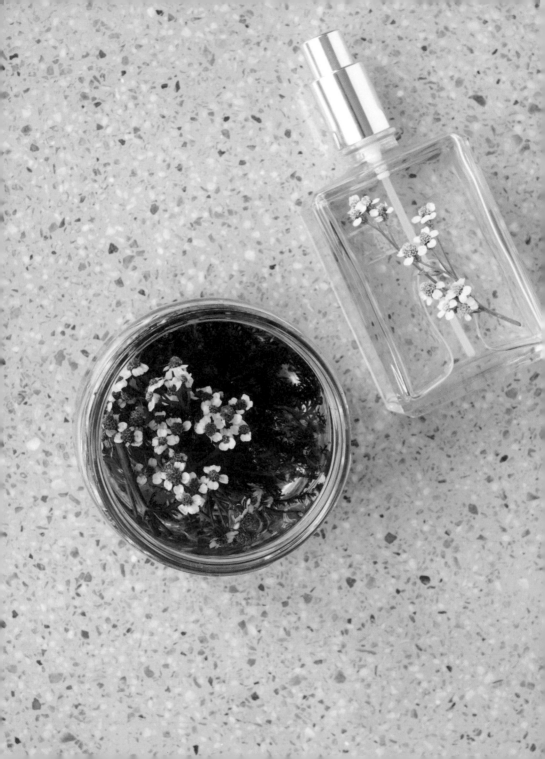

# YARROW SPRAY

Yarrow is a wonderful plant for your skin. It is restorative and helps wounds to heal, so I like to have it in spray form to apply it to minor wounds. Yarrow spray is also effective if you suffer from acne or other skin imperfections.

### Ingredients for 200ml

- 25–50g yarrow flowers and leaves (enough to fill the pot)
- 175ml vodka
- Spring water
- A clean 200ml pot or jar with lid
- A clean 200ml spray bottle

Fill the pot to the top with the leaves and flowers, then pour over the vodka to cover the plant material. Put the lid on the pot and add a label. Leave to stand for six weeks, then strain and the yarrow tincture is ready for use. Decant the tincture into the spray bottle and top up with spring water in the ratio of one third tincture, two thirds spring water.

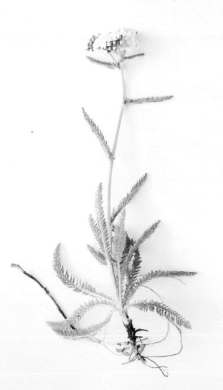

# ST JOHN'S WORT
(Hypericum perforatum)

Hypericaceae

## Effect on the skin
Disinfectant, soothing and helps wounds heal.

## When to use
On surgical wounds, deep wounds, burns, sunburn, scarring, inflamed wounds and breakouts (dab on undiluted tincture).

## Active ingredients
Hypericin, hyperforin, flavonoids, phenolic acid, tannins, bitter substances, essential oil, resin and vitamins A, B and C.

## Use

Flowering tips for the tincture. You can use the tincture undiluted as iodine.

Flowers for the oil. The amount of red pigments in the flowers is at its highest around 24 June. Harvest the flowers with the red stamens. You can use the oil in its pure state or as a base for ointments. You can also take it internally: one teaspoon on an empty stomach for nervous tension and stomach cramps.

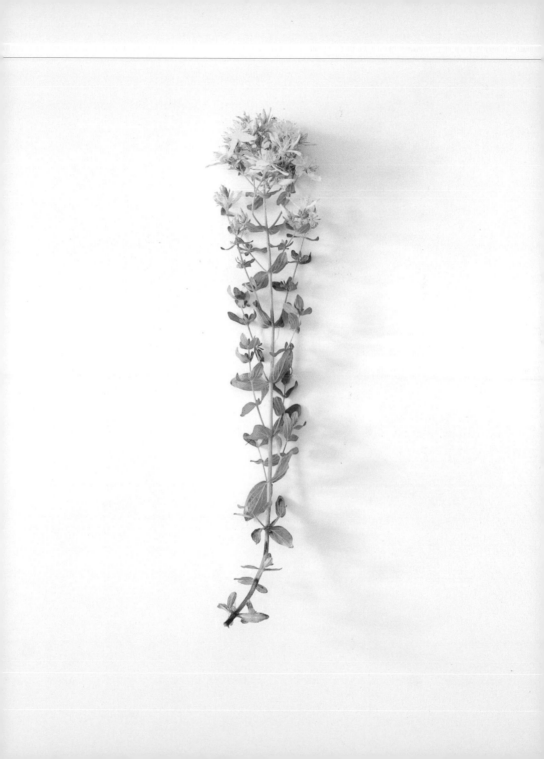

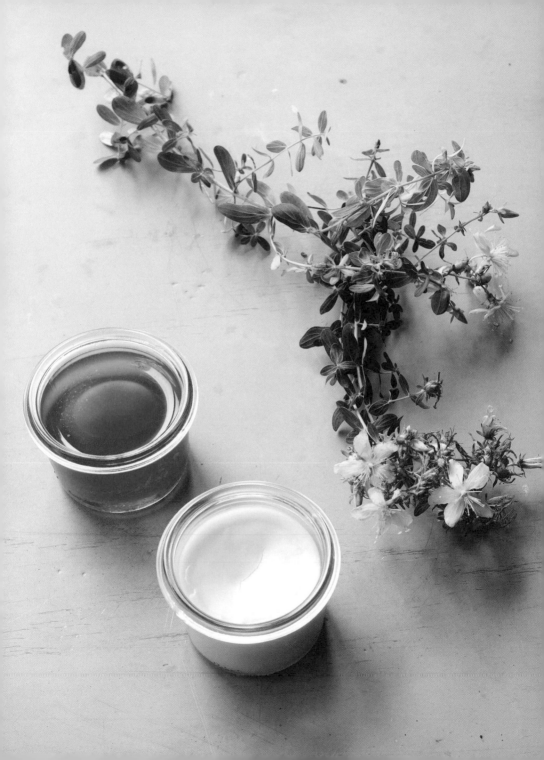

# ST JOHN'S OIL

St John's wort is a true rescue remedy; it is disinfectant, helps wounds heal, soothes sunburn, open wounds, surgical wounds, deep wounds and superficial burns.

## Ingredients for 200ml
- Approx. 50–100g fresh St John's wort flowers – only use the beautiful fully yellow flowers with a visible centre (enough to fill the pot)
- Approx. 175ml good-quality sunflower, olive or almond oil (enough to cover the flowers)
- A clean 200ml pot with lid
- Muslin

Fill the pot with the flowers (including the stamens) and pour the oil over them until it reaches the top of the pot. Make sure that the flowers are completely covered. Mix to remove any air bubbles, then cover with muslin and an elastic band. Leave to stand for two to four weeks in a sunny spot, stirring briefly on a daily basis. Strain and the marvellous red oil is ready for use.

# PINK OINTMENT WITH ST JOHN'S OIL

You can apply this ointment to rashes, sunburn and cold sores.

## Ingredients for 120g
- 20g beeswax
- 100ml St John's oil (see left)
- A clean 120ml pot with lid

Melt the beeswax in a water bath. Add the St John's oil, mix thoroughly and pour into the pot. Leave to set and then put the lid on the pot.

## Other tips for sunburn
Place cucumber slices on or apply pure aloe vera to the sunburnt skin.

71

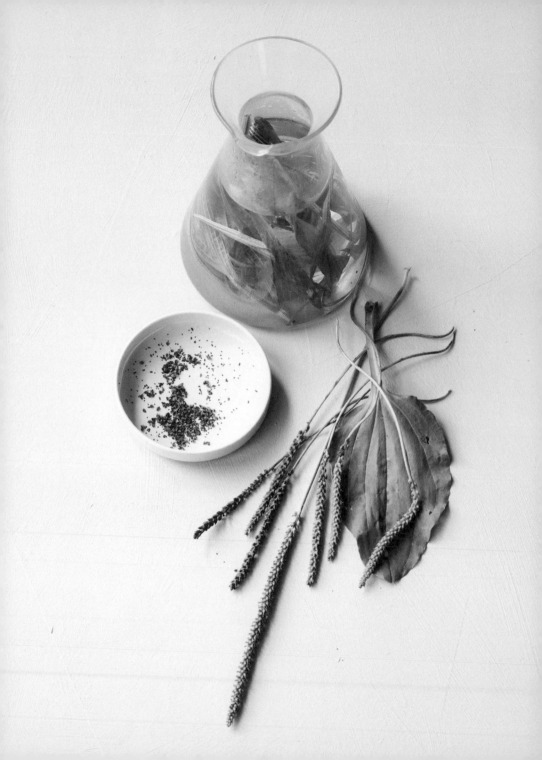

# RIBWORT PLANTAIN AND BROADLEAF PLANTAIN

(Plantago lanceolata and Plantago major)

Plantaginaceae


Both types of plantain have a medicinal effect on the skin.

## Effect on the skin
The leaves encourage blood clotting and help wounds to heal. They can be applied directly to the skin. The seeds are anti-inflammatory.

## When to use
On bloody wounds as well as cuts and abrasions. On insect bites, allergic skin reactions and inflamed skin.

## Active ingredients
Tannins, minerals including sulphur, iron, potassium, calcium, phosphorus, sodium, silicon and zinc, vitamins C and choline, glycoside aucubin, xanthophyll, resin, bitter substances, organic acids and alkaloids. Mucilage in the seeds.

## Use
Leaves of the ribwort plantain when in flower for a tincture. You can use the tincture to make a spray to ward off insect bites or apply it with a compress.
Mature leaves for a tea. Dry the leaves quickly, touching them as little as possible, then snip into rough pieces. You can use plaintain tea for a compress.
The seeds of the rosette-forming plantain are rich in mucilage (even greater than linseed) and can be used as a paste to treat skin inflammation — just like the seeds of fellow plantain family member psyllium (*Plantago psyllium*).

# PLANTAIN OINTMENT

Use plantain ointment on bloody wounds, poorly healing wounds, bruises, broken blood vessels (rosacea), allergic rashes and poor circulation. For the ointment, start by making a plantain oil as the base.

### Ingredients for 200ml oil
- 25–50g plantain leaves (enough to fill the pot)
- Approx. 175ml organic olive or sunflower oil (enough to cover the leaves
- A clean 200ml pot or jar with lid
- Muslin

Harvest the young, tender plantain leaves on a dry day in the late morning (once the dew has dried). Rub lightly or leave them on a cloth to dry. Snip them into small pieces and fill the pot to just below the top. Pour over oil to the top of the pot, then cover with muslin and an elastic band. Leave to stand in a light spot for approximately four weeks, stirring occasionally, then strain the oil.

### Ingredients for 120ml ointment
- 20g beeswax
- 100ml plantain oil
- Optional: 10 drops essential oil of your choice to fragrance the ointment

- A clean 125ml pot or jar with lid

Put the beeswax in a small dish, place the dish in the water bath and heat. Once the wax is melted, add the plantain oil and mix thoroughly. Add the essential oil, if using, mix thoroughly and pour into the ointment pot. Leave to cool and set, then put the lid on the pot and label it.

**TIP**
You can use the same procedure to make yarrow ointment.

# PLANTAIN JUICE FROM BOILED LEAVES

This juice soothes irritated skin, breakouts and sunburn.

### Ingredients for approximately 120ml
- 20g (10 leaves) rosette-forming or ribwort plantain
- 150ml water

Put the leaves in a small pan with the water, bring to the boil and cook for 5 minutes. Leave to cool and then apply the juice to the affected skin. The juice has a maximum shelf life of 2 days.

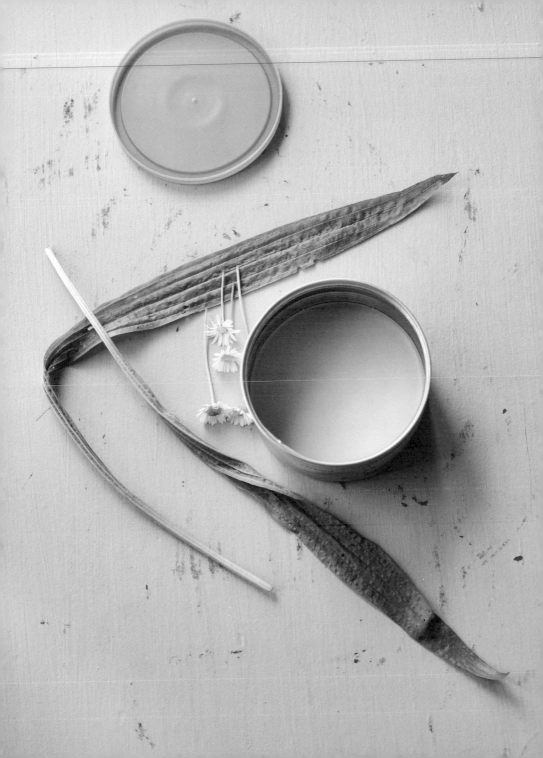

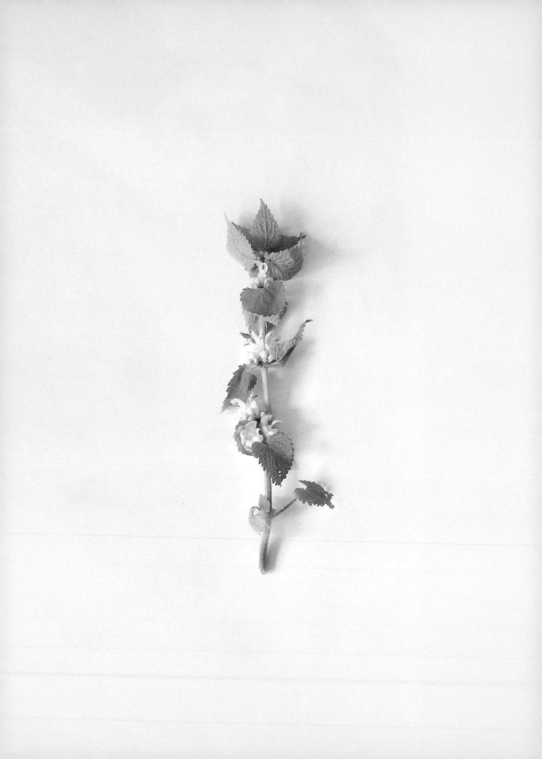

# WHITE DEADNETTLE

(Lamium album)

Lamiaceae

The deadnettle often grows in the vicinity of the common nettle and looks very similar; the only difference is that the deadnettle has white lipped flowers and does not sting. You can also use it to soothe stings from common nettles by rubbing the leaves over the affected skin to reduce the burning sensation.

## Effect on the skin
Soothes skin and encourages wound healing (because the plant contains xanthophyll).

## When to use
On minor wounds and patches of dry eczema, as well as skin that has come into contact with stinging nettles.

## Active ingredients
Mucilage, tannins, essential oil, bitter substances, saponins, choline, high levels of vitamin C, xanthophyll, histamine and potassium.

## Use
Fresh leaves and flowering tips for an infusion or tincture, as well as in soups and salads.
Flowering tips for a tea. The tips can take quite a long time to dry.

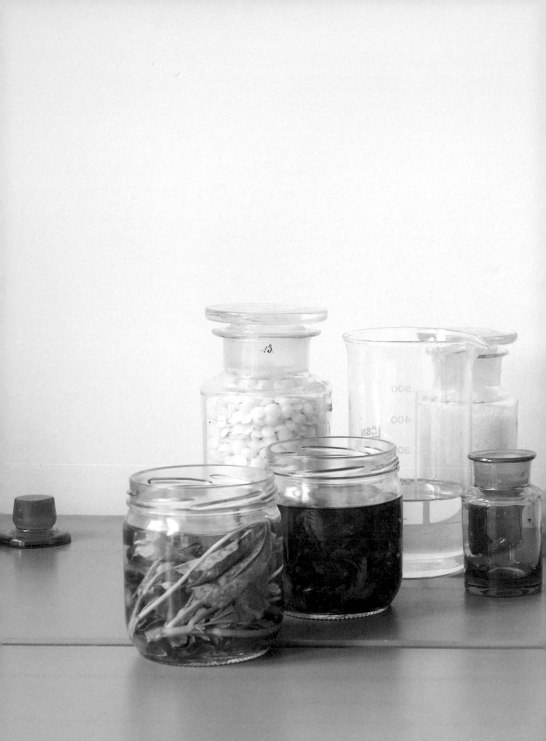

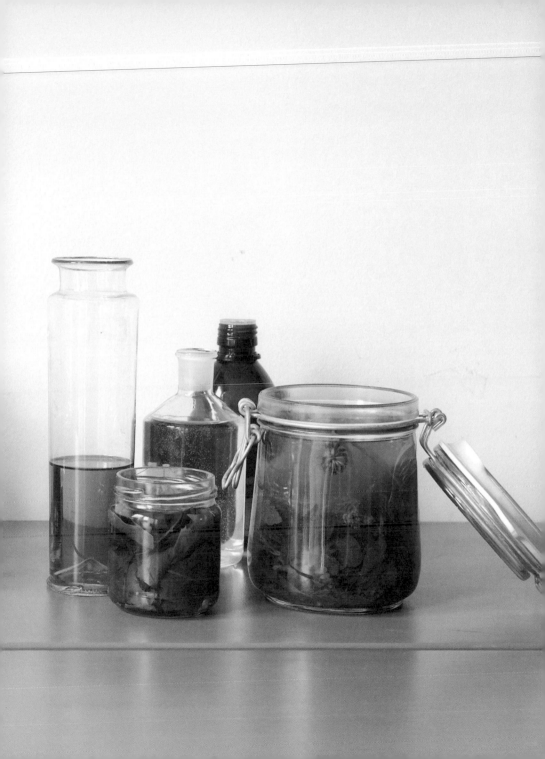

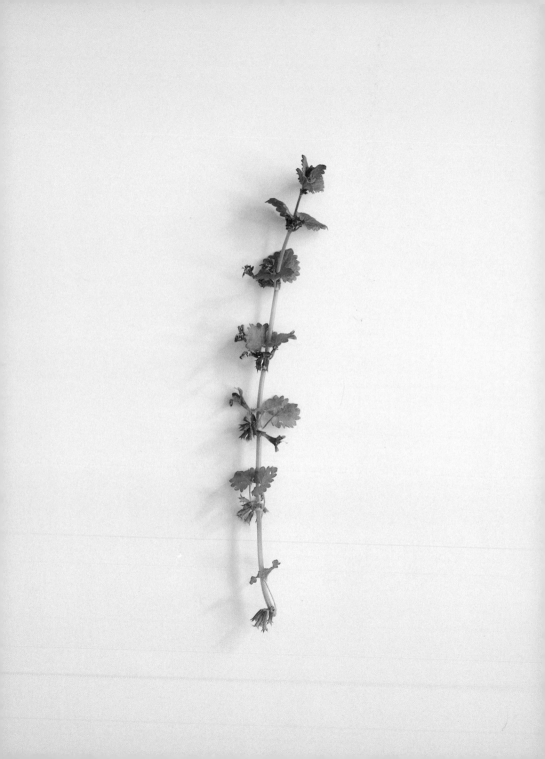

# GROUND IVY
(Glechoma hederacea)

Lamiaceae

Ground ivy used to be known as field balm as well, as it is useful for treating minor wounds; simply chew a leaf and use the resulting paste to cover the wound. Ground ivy oil is also very useful for treating earache, for example. Simply spread the oil around the painful area (for external use).

## When to use
On insect bites and nettle stings, inflammation and poorly healing wounds.

## Active ingredients
Bitter substances (glechomin), tannins, essential oil, organic acids, saponins, vitamin c and choline, as well as the minerals potassium, calcium and silicon.

## Use
The flowering plant (leaves and flowers) for a tincture, oil or tea.
Pick fresh leaves in spring for an infusion or in salads, or use them to make pesto.

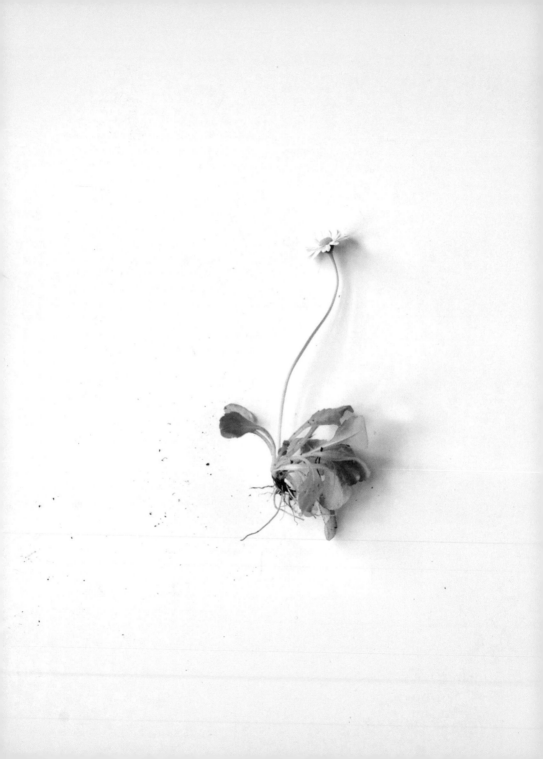

# DAISY
## (Bellis perennis)

Asteraceae

The daisy is a wonderful plant for your skin. Use it to make an oil or ointment to treat rashes and childhood diseases like chickenpox that involve skin blemishes.

## Effect on the skin
Soothes pain and itching and is both anti-inflammatory and antibacterial.

## When to use
On haematomas, bruising and poorly healing wounds. For childhood diseases that involve breakouts, including rubella, measles, roseola and chickenpox. Use as a skin wash or on a compress for rashes.

## Active ingredients
Saponins, mucilage, tannins, bitter substances, flavonol glycosides, essential oil, vitamin C, calcium, magnesium, organic acids and inulin.

## Use
Flowers with stems and leaves for a tincture. Use diluted tincture on a compress: add 40 drops tincture to 1 litre boiled, cooled water.
Flowers for a tea or infusion.
Leave flowers to infuse in a base oil to make an infused oil (see pages 12-13).

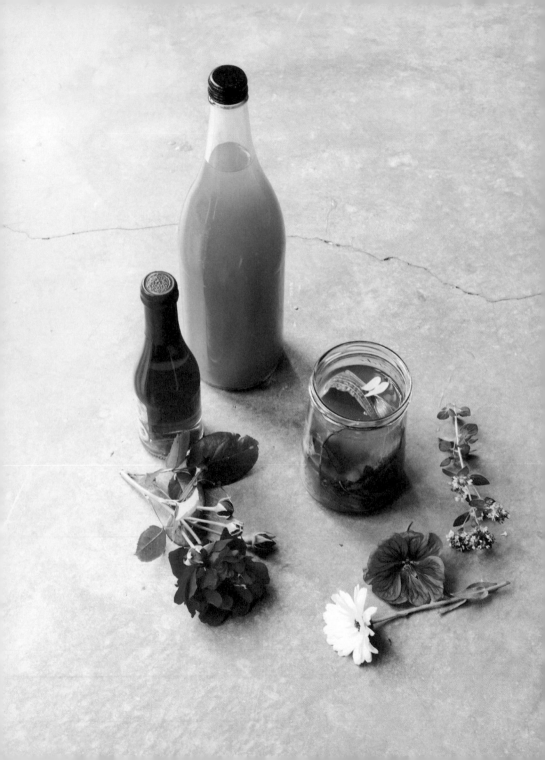

# QUEEN OF HUNGARY'S WATER

This is a very old recipe that is still used to make a tonic for your face. Back in 1300, an alchemist created the tonic for the Queen of Hungary so that she would stay looking youthful. An alternative story is that this recipe originated with travelling nomads. This wonderful face toner is pH neutral, is soothing and calming for your skin, and minimizes the appearance of your pores. It also softens and nourishes your hair.

## Ingredients for approximately 200ml

- 6g lemon balm
- 4g camomile flowers
- 4g rose petals
- 3g marigolds
- 3g common comfrey leaves
- 1g rosemary leaves
- Zest of half an organic lemon
- 175ml apple cider vinegar
- 100ml rose distillate or witch hazel hydrolate
- A clean 200ml pot or jar with lid

Place all the plant parts in the pot along with the lemon zest. Pour over the apple cider vinegar to cover the plant parts. Put the lid on the pot and leave to stand at room temperature for three to four weeks. Strain and then mix the vinegar (the extract) with the rose distillate or witch hazel hydrolate in a 1:1 ratio. In other words, if your pot has a capacity of 200ml, then add 100ml extract and 100ml distillate/hydrolate.

If the slightly sour fragrance of apple cider vinegar doesn't appeal to you, then omit it and just use rose distillate or witch hazel hydrolate. Store in a cool, dark place.

If you want to use the tonic as a face toner, decant it into an atomizer and spray on your skin daily, either in the morning or evening.

# REJUVENATING FACE OIL

This oil is the ideal choice if your skin is dry or more mature.

## Ingredients for approximately 200ml
- 50ml moringa oil
- 50ml jojoba oil
- 3g stinging nettle or field horsetail leaves
- 3g marigolds
- 3g camomile flowers
- 3g hibiscus flowers
- 100ml rosehip oil
- Muslin
- A clean 200ml dark bottle with cap

You can also choose just one oil and use 200ml of that.

## Optional
- 20 drops essential rose oil
- 20 drops vitamin E oil

Place the moringa and jojoba oils in a glass dish with the dry plant parts, place the dish in a water bath and heat for approximately 48 hours. Turn the heat off at night and on again the next morning, so you can monitor it consistently. Leave the oil to cool and then strain through muslin, squeezing out the plant parts. Add the rosehip oil, along with the rose and vitamin E oils (if using).

Mix thoroughly, pour into the bottle and close with the cap.

# CLEANSING YOUR FACE

There are different ways to cleanse your skin; you can give yourself a steam bath or use a home-made cleanser, a hydrolate or an infusion of flowers or plants.

# HERBAL STEAM BATHS

Steam baths are a wonderful way to cleanse your skin. They open your pores and clean them out, then you can use a (diluted) hydrolate to close them again. I prefer to use camomile in my steam baths, but you can also use other flowers or twigs, including rose, eucalyptus, pine or lavender.

Whatever you choose, place the plant parts in a bowl and pour hot water over them. Sit with your face above the bowl and put a towel over your head, to stop the steam from escaping and direct it onto the skin of your face. Enjoy your steam bath for approximately 20 minutes, or two five-minute sessions with a quick cool down in between.

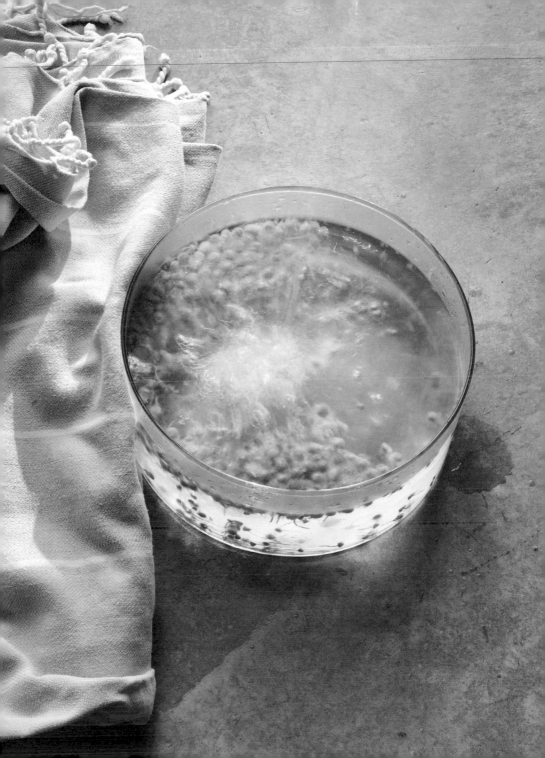

# CATCHWEED
## (Galium aparine)

Rubiaceae

Catchweed or cleavers 'catches hold' of your body's waste materials and carries them away. You can use it both externally and internally.

## Effect on the skin
Cleansing and tissue regenerating.

## When to use
On blemished skin, eczema, psoriasis, ulcers and wounds. Also effective for arthritis.

## Active ingredients
Bitter iridoids, organic acids, tannins, coumarins, red pigment and flavanoids.

## Use
Twigs, leaves and flowers for a tincture, tea or infusion.

# ICE CUBES WITH CATCHWEED AND ALOE VERA

These ice cubes are cooling and soothing for your skin.

## Ingredients for 12 ice cubes
• A handful of catchweed (cleavers)
• 50ml water
• 50ml aloe vera gel

Put the catchweed (cleavers) in the blender with the water and aloe vera gel and blend thoroughly. Transfer the mixture to an ice cube tray and leave in the freezer for 12 hours.

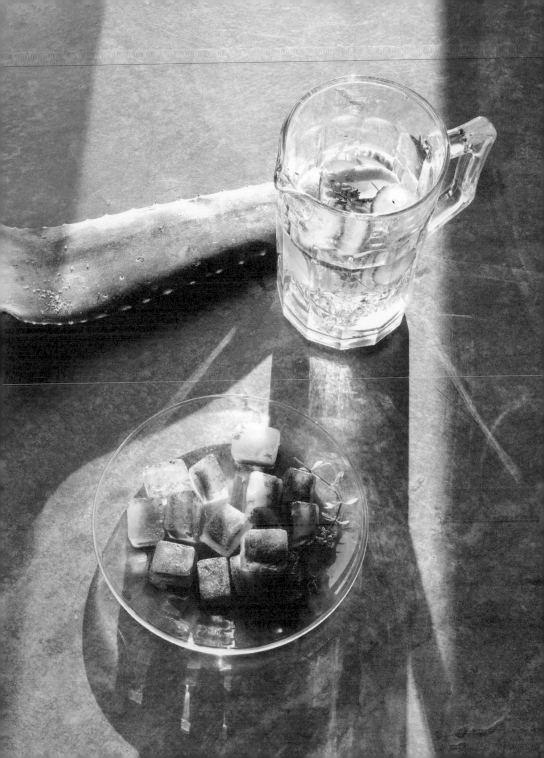

# HIBISCUS
(Hibiscus)

Malvaceae

Hibiscus is a common ingredient in beauty products. The plant is a member of the mallow family and is equally beneficial for your skin and hair. Hibiscus is nourishing and hydrating, protects your skin against premature ageing and gives your hair a wonderful glossy shine. You can use both fresh and dried flowers.

# MALLOW, COMMON
(Malva sylvestris)

Malvaceae

Mallow is soothing and calming for your skin.

## Effect on the skin
Soothes inflamed skin and helps to bring boils, sores and abscesses to a head and drain the contents.

## When to use
On inflamed skin, psoriasis and patches of dry eczema. Use both internally and externally.

## Use
The flowers and leaves.
Make an infusion or maceration by leaving flowers to infuse in cold water and then heating it slowly. Turn off the heat before the water comes to the boil.
Fresh leaves: add them to your smoothie or press to extract the juice.

# INFUSION OF HIBISCUS (OR MALLOW)

An infusion of hibiscus is wonderfully nourishing and hydrating for your skin and hair, plus the flower turns the water a beautiful pink colour.

Place a handful of dried flowers in a jug, pour boiled water over them and leave to cool. Use to cleanse and nourish your skin or as a rinse for your hair. You can also use mallow, but make sure that you leave the flowers to infuse in cold water first before heating slowly.

# MASKS

There are lots of ways to make masks — you can use products from your pantry and kitchen cupboards, for example, or harvest plants growing in your neighbourhood. You can make masks from a range of ingredients, including clay, fruit pulp, oil, hydrolates and apple cider vinegar.

## CLEANSING FACE MASK

This wonderful mask contains aloe vera, kaolin clay and olive oil.

**Ingredients for 1 mask**
• 10g aloe vera
• 10g (1 tbsp) kaolin clay (powder)
• 1 tsp olive oil

Mix the ingredients thoroughly and apply as a face mask. Leave for 20 minutes and rinse off with tepid water.

## THREE QUICK AND EASY MASKS

Each of the following masks uses just two ingredients; 1 teaspoon of each. Simply mix them together and your mask is ready to apply.

**Ingredients for 1 astringent mask**
• 5g (1 tsp) red clay
• 1 tsp rosewater

**Ingredients for 1 nourishing mask**
• 5g (1 tsp) white bentonite clay
• 1 tsp witch hazel hydrolate

**Ingredients for 1 cleansing mask**
• 5g (1 tsp) Dead Sea mud or powder
• 1 tsp apple cider vinegar

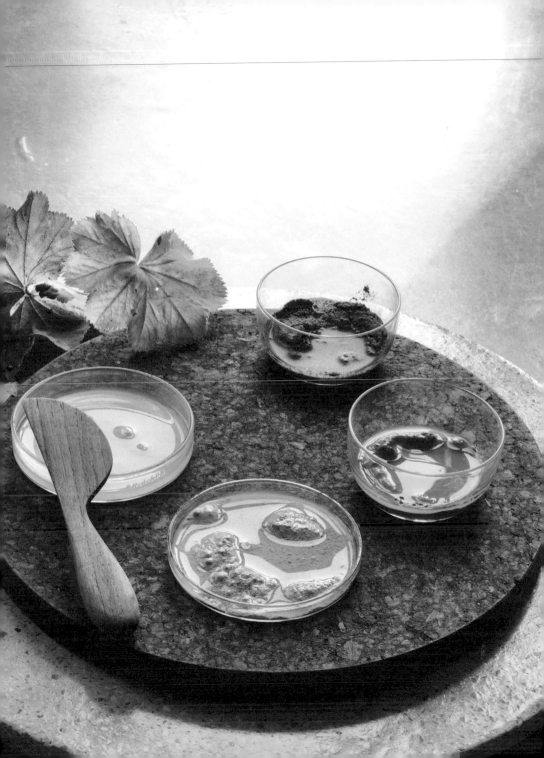

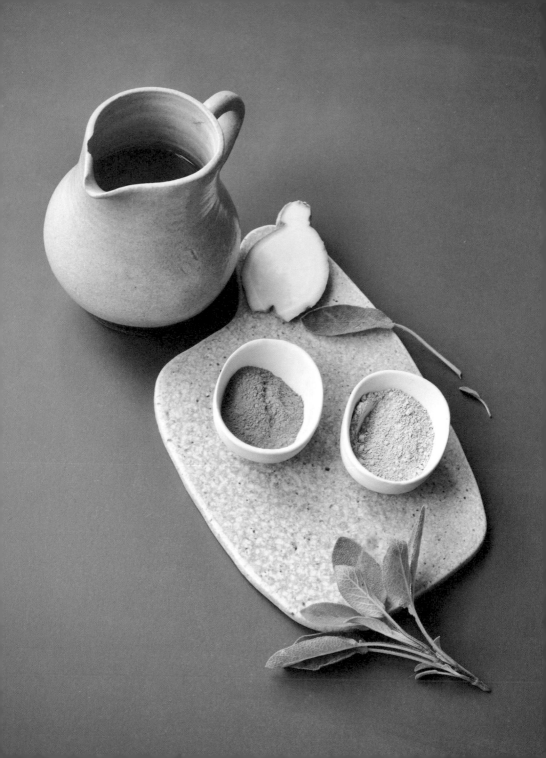

# NOURISHING MASKS

## FACE MASK WITH GINGER AND TURMERIC

Curcumin, a substance in turmeric, is a powerful anti-inflammatory, which is why turmeric can help treat acne or skin breakouts. Curcumin is also an antioxidant, it helps to reduce wrinkles and pigmentation marks, and encourages wounds and bruises to heal.

### Ingredients for 1 mask
- 2 tsp honey
- 1 tsp lemon juice
- 1 tsp grated ginger
- ½ tsp turmeric powder or grated turmeric

Mix the ingredients thoroughly and apply the mask either to your entire face (avoiding the area around your eyes) or simply to areas where you have blemishes. Leave for 10 minutes and then rinse off with tepid water.

## FACE MASK WITH CARROT

This mask is effective against skin imperfections and premature aging.

### Ingredients for 1 mask
- 2 small carrots
- 10ml (1 tsp) almond or olive oil

Cook the carrots until they have softened, then mash them and add the almond or olive oil. Apply the mask to your face, leave for 20 to 30 minutes and rinse off with tepid water.

--

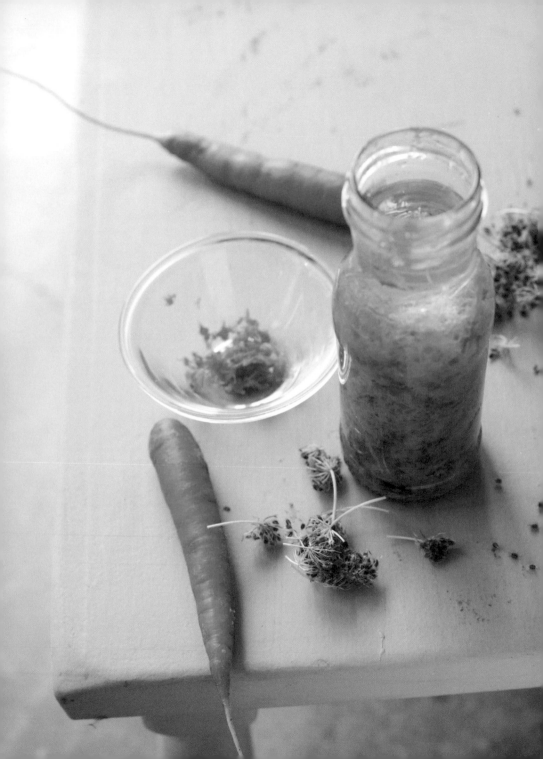

# CARROT SKIN OIL

Carrots are packed with vitamins and minerals that nourish and protect your skin.

**Ingredients for 150ml**
- 2 carrots
- 100ml good-quality oil
- A clean 150ml pot or jar
- Muslin
- A clean 150ml bottle with cap

Wash and grate the carrots, then place them in the pot and pour over the oil. Cover with muslin and leave for four weeks, stirring occasionally. Strain the oil through muslin and pour into the bottle.

You can recongize wild carrot from the 'lace skirt' below the flower. That's why the plant is also referred to as 'Queen Anna's lace'.

**TIP**
Wild carrot (*Daucus carota*) is the ancestor of the cultivated carrot we know today. You can press a wonderful oil from the seeds of the wild carrot, or leave the seeds in oil to infuse (macerate).

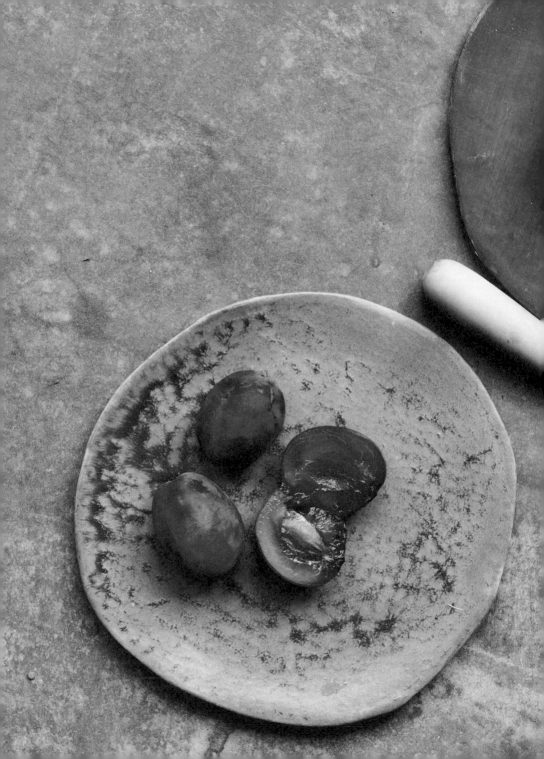

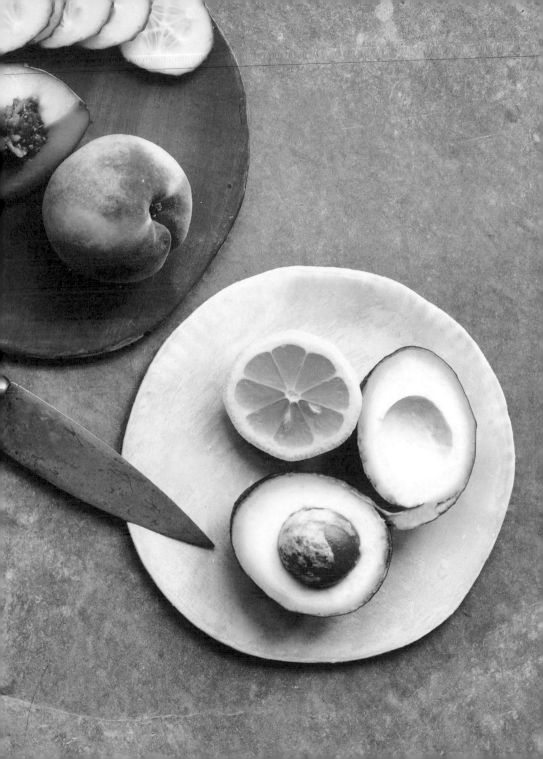

# FACE MASK WITH AVOCADO AND LEMON

Lemon juice contains vitamin C, which not only stops the avocado from turning brown as quickly but also has an astringent and slightly dehydrating effect. That's welcome if your skin is oily, but less so if it's dry. The oil balances out the dehydrating effect of the lemon juice somewhat, while the avocado is rich in unsaturated fats and nourishes your skin.

### Ingredients for 1 mask
- ½ avocado
- 1 tbsp lemon juice
- 1 tbsp olive oil

Mash the avocado and add the lemon juice and olive oil. Mix thoroughly and apply to your face as a mask. Leave for 20 to 30 minutes and rinse off with tepid water.

# FACE MASK WITH AVOCADO AND ALOE VERA

This is a wonderfully nourishing mask for drier skin.

### Ingredients for 1 mask
- ½ avocado
- 2 tbsp aloe vera gel
- 1 tbsp oatmeal
- 1 tbsp honey

Mash the avocado in a dish and add the aloe vera gel. Mix in the other ingredients and apply to your skin. Leave for approximately 20 minutes and rinse off with tepid water.

# PLUM MASK

# ROSEHIP MASK

Plums (*Prunus domestica*) are rich in vitamins A, C, E, K and B, antioxidants and iron, potassium and magnesium. They protect your skin cells and regulate the amount of sebum produced.

## Ingredients for 1 mask
- 2 plums
- 1 tbsp lemon juice
- 1 tbsp olive oil

Remove the stones from the plums and mash the flesh of the fruit. Stir in the lemon juice and olive oil and mix thoroughly. Apply to your face as a mask, leave for 20 to 30 minutes and rinse off with tepid water.

Rosehips are packed with vitamin C and other oxidants. Puree them and mix with a little water, then strain to remove the seeds. Apply the pulp to your skin, leave for 20 minutes and rinse off with tepid water.

## You can also use this method to make masks from:

- **Sea buckthorn** (*Hippophae rhamnoides*). Rich in vitamin C and other antioxidants.
- **Apricot** (*Prunus armeniaca*). The apricot's kernel (stone) contains essential oil. If you remove the kernel, you can puree the fresh fruit and apply it as a face mask to cleanse your skin and leave it silky soft.
- **Almond** (*Prunus dulcis*) You can also use almond flour and almond milk to make excellent face masks. Mix the almond flour with a dash of water, apply to your face and leave for 30 minutes. Or drip some organic almond milk on a cotton pad and dab onto your face. Leave overnight.

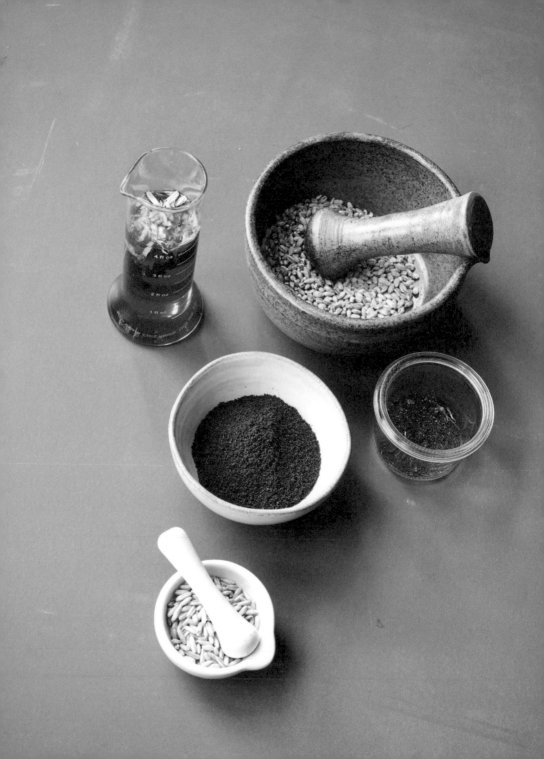

# SCRUBS

You can remove dead skin cells with a natural scrub made from ingredients like oats or barley. Grind them finely with a pestle and mortar — unless you are using coffee grounds, which are also an excellent choice, before adding a dash of water.

## FACE SCRUB WITH ROSEHIP OIL, SHEA BUTTER AND COFFEE GROUNDS

This nourishing scrub is a gentle yet effective way to remove dead surface skin cells.

### Ingredients for 50ml
- 50g shea butter
- 50ml rosehip oil
- 2 tbsp coffee grounds
- Optional: 10 drops essential oil of your choice
- A clean 50ml pot or jar with lid

Melt the shea butter in a small pan, add the rosehip oil and mix thoroughly. Then add the coffee grounds and essential oil (if using) and mix thoroughly. Transfer to the pot, put the lid on the pot and apply a label.

You can also replace the coffee grounds with the following ingredients:
- Oats, millet, barley or another type of grain, finely ground in a pestle and mortar
- 1 tbsp Himalayan sea salt
- Cane sugar

# USING SALICYLIC ACID ON THE SKIN

As I've already said, salicylic acid is effective if your skin is oily, blemished or irritated. Salicin — a natural component of meadowsweet and willow — is converted into salicylic acid. If you apply salicin (and thus salicylic acid) to your skin, it dissolves the sebum in your pores, so salicin treats breakouts, blackheads and styes.

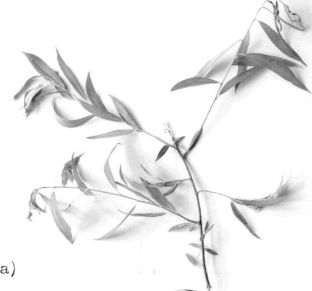

## WILLOW
(Salix alba)

Salicaceae

The bark of the white willow also contains the anti-inflammatory component salicin, which is effective against acne. You can use willow for shingles, nerve pain and nervous skin breakouts. Boil the bark for an infusion or make a tincture. Apply an infusion or diluted tincture to your skin.

# MEADOWSWEET
(Filipendula ulmaria)

Rosaceae

This plant is often found growing near water
and the flowers have a wonderful fragrance.
Meadowsweet is antiseptic and soothes your
skin.

## Effect on the skin
Astringent, nurturing, anti-inflammatory
and analgesic.

## When to use
On acne and skin imperfections, nerve
pain and nervous skin breakouts. Use
a compress with diluted tincture on
chickenpox, shingles and acne, or apply an
infusion or diluted tincture to your skin.

## Active ingredients
Essential oils, flavonoids, tannins,
mucilage, minerals including calcium,
iron, potassium, manganese, silicon,
phosphorus and sulphur. Vitamin C, organic
acids, glycosides and coumarins.

## Use
The root in spring; the flowers and leaves
in summer. For a double tincture, make a
tincture with the root in spring and then add
flowers and leaves in summer.
Flowering tips, stem and leaves for a tea or
infusion. You can also make a hydrolate from the
flowers and use it as an astringent, nurturing and
nourishing face tonic.

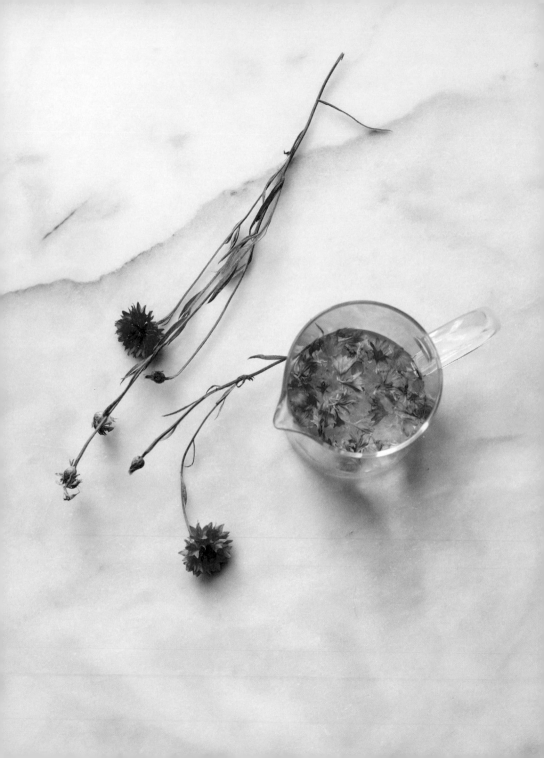

# LOOKING AFTER YOUR EYES

If your eyes are inflamed, try cleaning them with a cotton pad and some eyewash made with camomile or cornflower. Always use a separate clean pad for each eye and wipe carefully from the outer to the inner corner.

## EYEWASH WITH CAMOMILE

Camomile is soothing and anti-inflammatory.

**Ingredients**
- Approx. 5g (one handful) camomile flowers
- 100ml boiled water

Pour the water over the camomile, leave to cool and strain before using.

## EYEWASH WITH CORNFLOWER

This eyewash is wonderfully soothing for irritated and over-stimulated eyes.

**Ingredients**
- Approx. 5g (one handful) cornflower flowers
- 100ml boiled water

Pour the water over the cornflowers, leave to cool and strain before using.

## CORNFLOWER
(Centaurea cyanus)

Asteraceae

Cornflower is used for mild eye problems and inflammations including styes, inflamed eyelids and conjunctivitis. Contains mucilage, tannins, bitter substances and metalloanthocyanins (cyanin).

**TIP**
You can also use the common poppy on your eyes. Placing cotton pads soaked with a poppy infusion on your eyelids is an effective way to ease tired and irritated eyes.

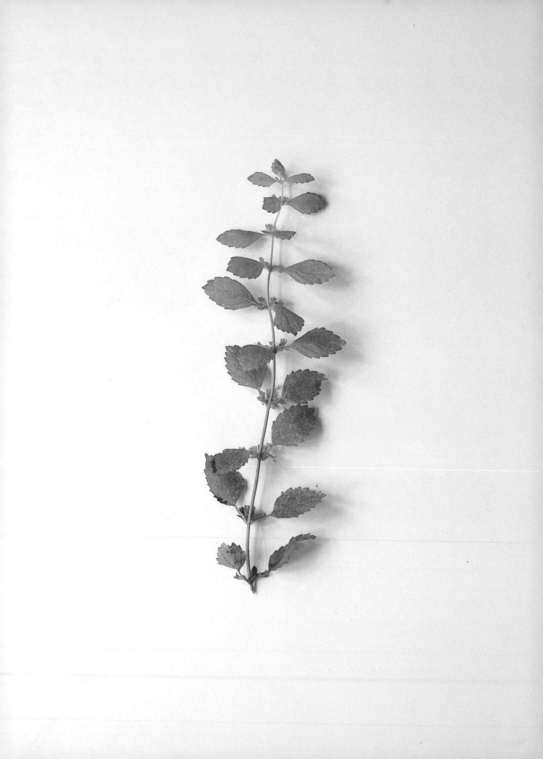

# LEMON BALM
## (Melissa officinalis)

Lamiaceae

Lemon balm is a wonderfully fragrant, lemony plant that is soothing for your skin. It has a disinfectant effect for viral skin infections such as cold sores and also repels midges and mosquitoes.

## Effect on the skin
Soothing, antiviral and repels midges and mosquitoes.

## When to use
On viral skin infections such as cold sores or shingles.

## Active ingredients
Essential oils, phenolic acids, tannins, bitter substances, mucilage, flavonoids, organic acids, vitamins C and E, and beta-carotene.

## Use
The leaves for a tincture. You can also use the flowers when the plant is in bloom.
The leaves for a tea. Dry them quickly and carefully, touching them as little as possible.
Fresh leaves for an infusion or in salads and smoothies.

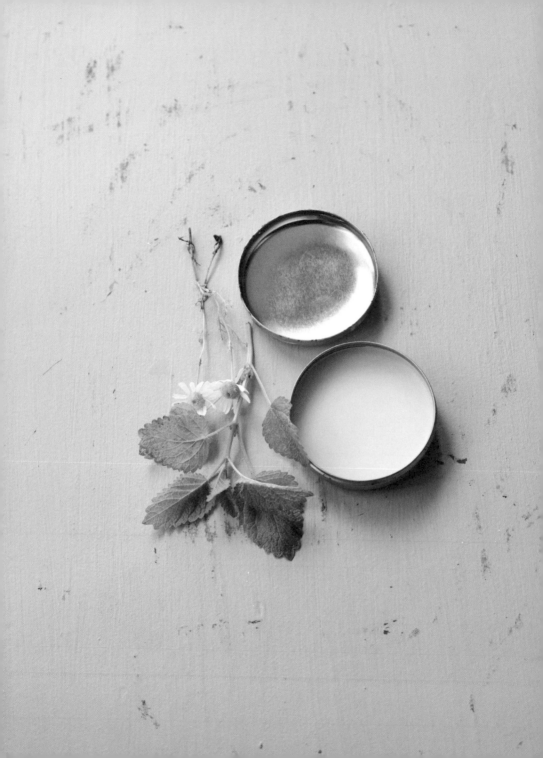

# LOOKING AFTER YOUR LIPS

## LIP BALM WITH LEMON BALM

This lip balm is cleansing and restorative if you have a cold sore or skin infection. The first step is to make an oil that you then use as a base for the lip balm.

### Ingredients for 200ml oil
- 50g lemon balm leaves, finely chopped
- 25g camomile flowers
- 175ml organic sunflower or olive oil
- A clean 200ml pot or jar with lid

Place the plant parts in the pot (until it is full), pour over the oil to cover them and cover the pot with a cotton cloth. Leave to stand for approximately four weeks, stirring occasionally, then strain the oil.

### TIP
You can also replace the lemon balm with camomile for a soothing lip balm.

### Ingredients for 100ml lip balm
- 20g beeswax
- 100ml lemon balm oil
- 10 drops essential lavender oil
- 5 drops vitamin E oil
- A clean 100ml pot or five 20ml ointment pots, with a lid or lids

Heat the beeswax in a water bath. Add the lemon balm oil and mix thoroughly. Add the essential oil and the vitamin E oil, mixing thoroughly. Decant into the pot or pots, leave to set and then add the lid or lids.

# LIP BALM WITH CAMOMILE

Wonderfully nourishing and soothing, particularly if you have chapped lips.

### Ingredients for 75ml
- 5g beeswax
- 60g shea butter
- 10ml camomile oil (oil that you have infused yourself, not essential oil)
- A clean 75ml pot with lid
- Muslin

Start by making the camomile oil. Place the flowers in a pot and cover with good-quality oil. Cover with muslin and leave to stand for four weeks, stirring regularly. Strain through muslin and the oil is ready for use.

### Then make the lip balm
Melt the beeswax in a water bath. Once the beeswax is melted completely, add the shea butter and mix thoroughly. Add the camomile oil, pour into a small pot, leave to set and then put the lid on the pot.

# JUNA'S LIP SCRUB

My 11-year-old daughter, Juna, makes herself a very effective yet simple lip scrub.

### Ingredients for approximately 10g
- 1 tbsp sugar
- 1 tsp honey
- A dash of olive oil (or replace the olive oil with a vegetable oil)
- A clean pot measuring 10ml, with lid

Mix the ingredients and transfer them to the pot. Freeze for a short period, then keep the lip scrub in the fridge.

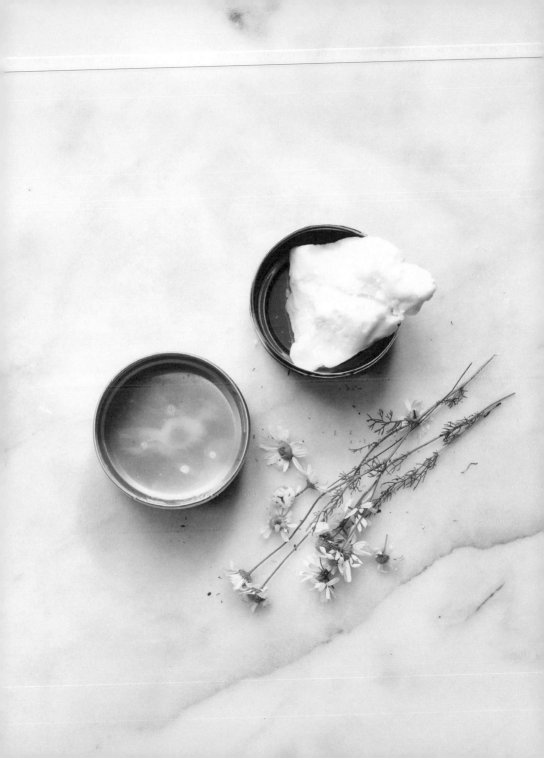

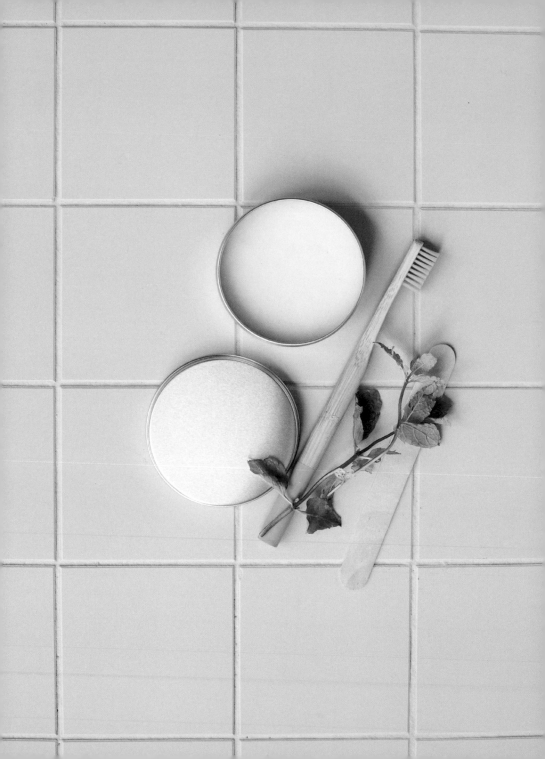

# LOOKING AFTER YOUR MOUTH

If you discovered that you'd run out of toothpaste, then you could also clean your teeth with coconut oil, baking soda or turmeric, as all three have antibacterial properties.

Baking soda neutralizes acids in your mouth, helps to remove plaque, and acts as a light abrasive to polish away any grey deposits on your teeth. To prevent your tooth enamel from being worn away, use no more than once a fortnight as toothpaste.

Making your own toothpaste is also quick and easy with ingredients including xylitol. This is a natural sweetener that helps to stop cavities forming and is also known as birch sugar.

## TOOTHPASTE

This toothpaste contains all the ingredients you need to look after your teeth properly.

### Ingredients for approximately 200g
- 100g calcium carbonate
- 80g baking soda
- 30g xylitol
- 15ml water
- 20 drops essential peppermint oil
- A clean 200g pot or jar with lid

Mix the dry ingredients thoroughly, add the water and then the essential oil. Continue mixing to form a paste and keep in the jar or pot.

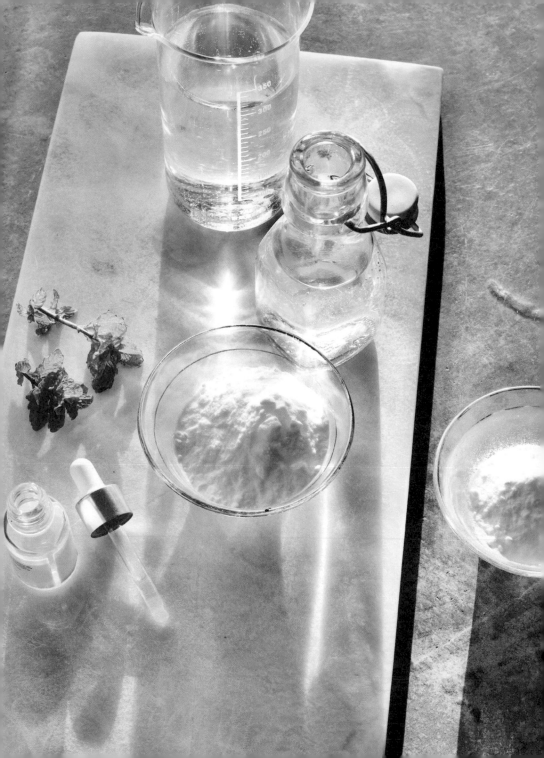

# MOUTHWASH AND OIL PULLING

Rinsing with mouthwash can be wonderfully refreshing. You can add various essential oils to add flavour and kill bacteria.

## Ingredients for approximately 100ml

- 5g (1 tsp) baking soda
- 5g xylitol
- 100ml filtered or boiled water at room temperature
- 10 drops essential oil (create a blend of your choice of peppermint, lemon, pine, tea tree, eucalyptus, fennel, aniseed and lavender)
- 1 drops essential clove oil
- Optional: 1 tbsp aloe vera gel
- A clean 100ml dark bottle with cap

Add the baking soda and xylitol to the water and mix thoroughly. Add the essential oils along with the aloe vera gel, if using, and transfer to a dark bottle. Shake well before using.

This mouthwash has a shelf life of approximately one week.

## Oil pulling: rinsing or cleaning with coconut oil

Rinsing your mouth with coconut oil - known as oil pulling - is a common Ayurvedic practice. Simply take a spoonful of coconut oil and swish it around your mouth for 20 minutes. Remember not to swallow it! After 20 minutes, spit out the oil and rinse with tepid water. Oil pulling boosts your metabolism, so your body can detox itself faster. The oil absorbs the bacteria in your mouth, so spitting it out cleanses your digestive system from your mouth to your bowels. Make sure to use a natural organic coconut oil, not one that has been stripped of its fragrance.

Another option is to clean your teeth with coconut oil, you can then choose to scrape your tongue clean with a spoon or tongue scraper.

# OATS
(Avena sativa)

Poaceae

Oats help with brittle nails and hair and are wonderfully soothing for your skin. Treat yourself all over with an oatmeal bath.

## Effect on the skin
Soothing and anti-inflammatory. Strengthens hair and nails.

## When to use
On itches, rashes, dry and rough skin, eczema and childhood diseases like chickenpox that involve rashes, as well as for brittle hair and nails. Can also help prevent tooth decay.

## Active ingredients
Starch, proteins, fats, sugars, mucilage, saponins, alkaloids, phytosterols, minerals including calcium, manganese, iron, phosphorus, silicon, potassium, copper, bromine and zinc, B vitamins (including folic acid), vitamins E and K.

## Use
The whole plant for a tincture. Harvest it immediately after flowering and before it sets fruit. The tincture is suitable for long-term use. Make an infusion by pouring hot, boiled water over the oats and leaving for four hours. Strain and apply the cool water to your skin or hair, or drink it to strengthen your skin, hair, teeth and nails from the inside out.

## TIP
Other grain types, including barley and rice, are also good for your skin and hair, as they are astringent and soothing. Make an infusion or strain, save and use the cooking water.

# COMMON IVY
(Hedera helix)

Araliaceae

You can use common ivy externally
to treat sores and poorly healing
wounds, arthritis, osteoarthritis,
muscle pain, sciatica, nerve pain,
superficial burns, sunburn, rashes and
head lice. Components in common ivy
include saponins, which are cleansing,
antibacterial and antifungal.

## IVY WATER

**Ingredients for 500ml**
• 50g ivy leaves
• 500ml cold water

Place the leaves and
water in a blender and
blend thoroughly.
Apply the mixture
directly to your skin
or make a compress
and place that on
your skin.

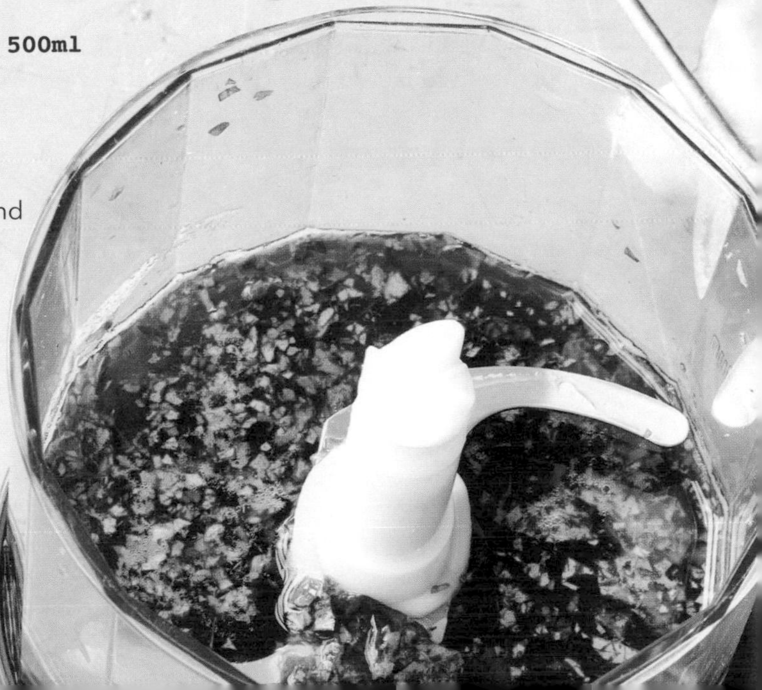

# LOOKING AFTER YOUR HAIR

Shop-bought shampoo tends to be harsh and aggressive and remove beneficial scalp oils, so you can benefit from making your own — either liquid or in bar form. You can also make your own conditioner with coconut milk or apple cider vinegar, or use infusions of nettle or field horsetail to give yourself stronger hair.

## LIQUID SHAMPOO

This is a basic recipe for a gentle shampoo.

### Ingredients for approximately 150ml
- 60ml coconut milk
- 80ml Castile soap
- 5ml olive oil
- 20 drops essential oil
- 5 drops vitamin E oil
- A clean 150ml pot or jar with lid

Gently heating the ingredients will help them to mix more thoroughly. Start by heating the coconut milk, then add the Castile soap and finally the olive oil, essential oil and vitamin E oil.

Mix thoroughly and pour into a bottle. Shake well before using.

### TIPS
Add a camomile infusion to the shampoo if you want to lighten your hair slightly. Or add a few drops of essential tea tree oil if you (or your child) unexpectedly catch head lice. Alternatively, you can add the tea tree oil to your conditioner and leave it on your hair for a while to work its magic.

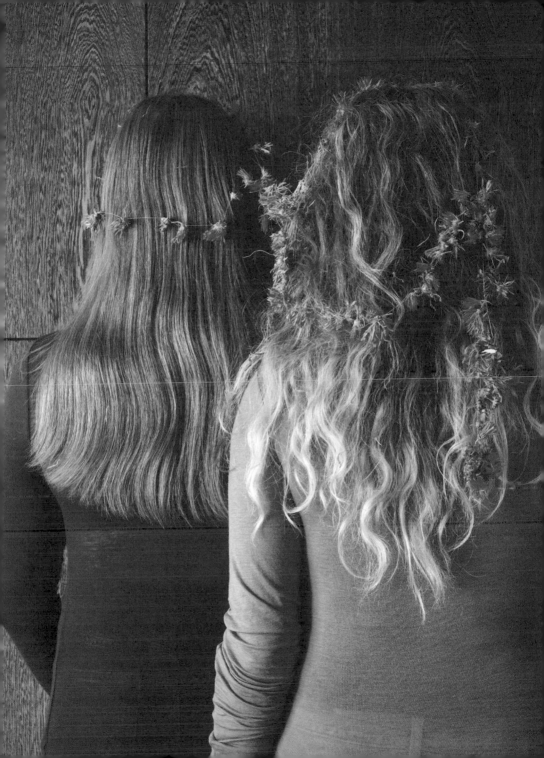

# SOLID SHAMPOO

If you buy a bottle of shampoo, you are mainly paying for water (80%), so both the environment and your wallet will benefit if you make a shampoo bar – essentially a piece of shampoo.

### Ingredients for 1 bar
• 50g sodium coco sulphate
• 10ml boiled water
• 8g coconut oil
• 4g shea butter
• Silicone mould for soap bars

### Optional
• 10 drops lavender oil
• 10 drops tea tree oil
• 10 drops argan oil

Heat the sodium coco sulphate and the boiled water in a water bath. Although it won't melt completely, it will form a sticky mass. Add the coconut oil and shea butter and mix thoroughly. Once everything has melted and mixed properly, remove the pan from the heat. Add the essential oils (if using) and/ or any other ingredients of your choice. Transfer the mixture to the silicone mould, then freeze for a short period, so that the shampoo sets more quickly. Remove the bar from the mould and leave to cure for another two days.

# DRY SHAMPOO

Sometimes you simply don't have the time to wash your hair and that's when this dry shampoo comes into its own.

### Ingredients for 120g
• 50g (3 tbsp) baking soda
• 30g (4 tbsp) arrowroot powder
• 30g (3 tsp) white clay powder
• 10 drops essential oil of your choice
• A clean 120g shaker

Mix all the ingredients thoroughly and put the mixture into the shaker.

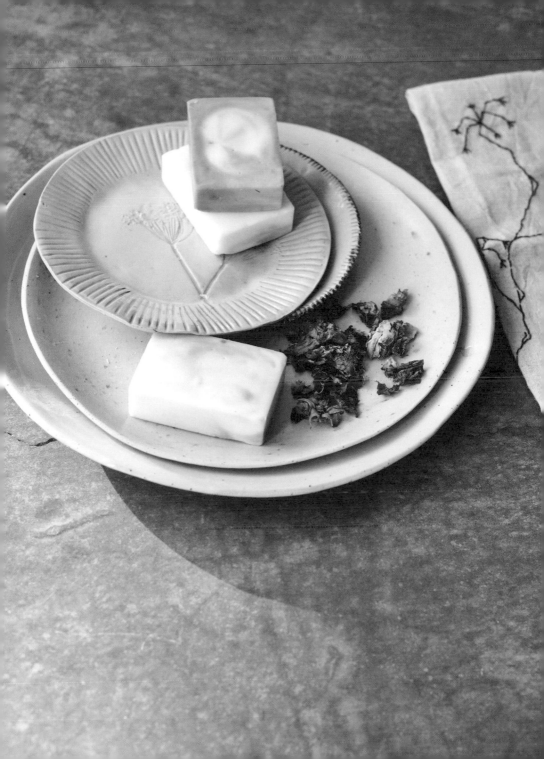

# CONDITIONERS FOR YOUR HAIR

There are plenty of products out there that can improve the condition of your hair, including these conditioners:

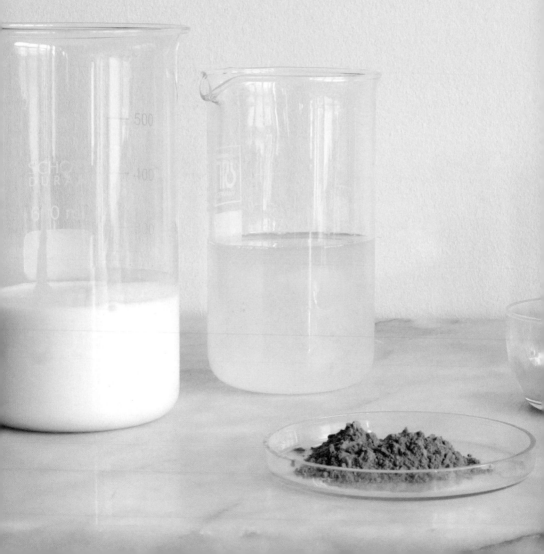

# APPLE CIDER VINEGAR WITH HERBS

Apple cider vinegar will nourish your hair and you can add plants like camomile, rosemary, thyme, common nettle, field horsetail and ground ivy to make a particularly effective conditioner.

**Ingredients for 150ml**
- 50–100g plant parts (enough to fill the pot)
- 150ml apple cider vinegar
- A clean 150ml pot or jar with lid

Fill the pot with the plant parts and pour over the apple cider vinegar to cover them. Leave to infuse for at least two weeks, then strain and your conditioner is ready for use.

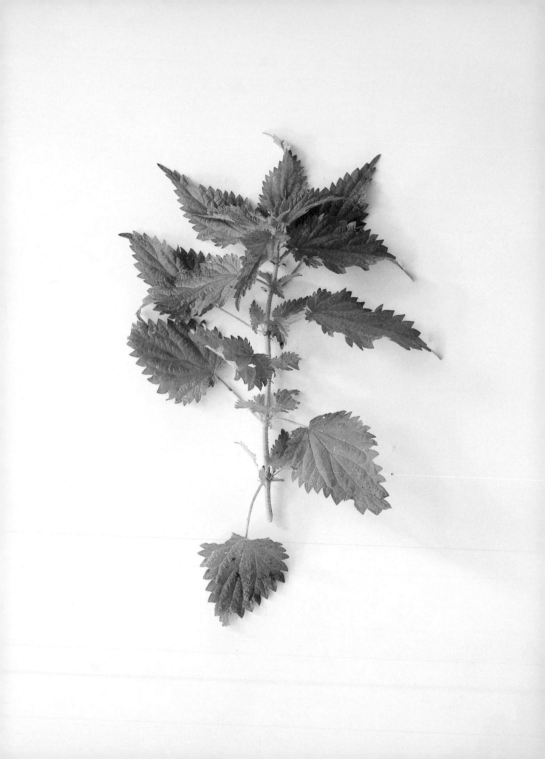

# COMMON NETTLE
(Urtica dioica and Urtica urens)

Urticaceae

Although the common nettle has a bad reputation because it delivers a painful, burning sting if you touch it, the plant is also very good for your skin. You can take it internally for acne, eczema or psoriasis; alternatively, rinsing with nettle water will help to cleanse dirty wounds and nourish your skin and hair.

## Effect on the skin and hair
Cleansing, detoxifying and deacidifying. It is also an effective tonic for your hair and scalp.

## When to use
Externally on dirty wounds, rashes, acne, boils and sores. As a tonic for your hair and scalp. Internally for acne, brittle nails and weakened cartilage.

## Active ingredients
Tannins, vitamins A, B, C, D, E and K, minerals including potassium, calcium, silicon, iron, sodium, magnesium, sulphur, chlorine, phosphorus, manganese, organic acids (including formic acid), chlorophyll, bitter substances, saponins, xanthophyll and histamine.

## Use
The young plant tips.

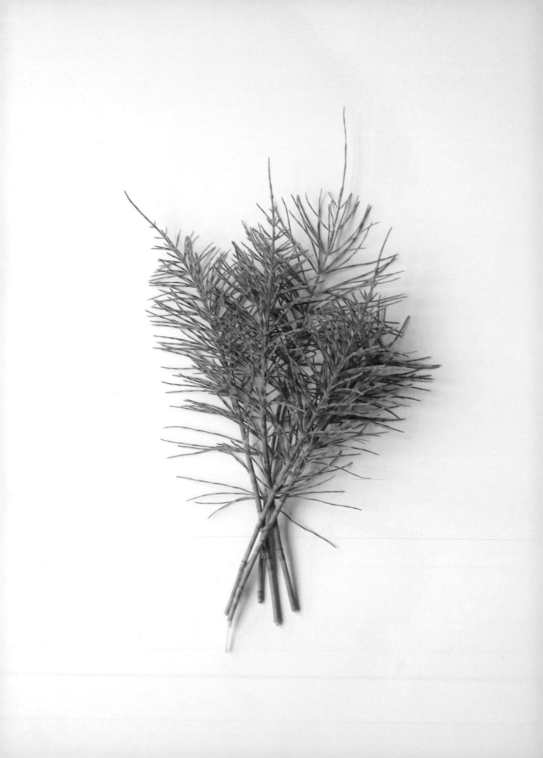

# FIELD HORSETAIL
(Equisetum arvense)

Equisetaceae

Field horsetail is packed with minerals and is rich in silicon; a trace element that strengthens your hair, nails and bones. Always harvest field horsetail from clean environments as the plant absorbs toxins from the soil.

## Effect on the skin and hair
Strengthens nails and hair, healing for your skin.

## When to use
For brittle nails and hair, poorly healing wounds, piles and contusions.

## Active ingredients
Minerals including silicon, calcium, potassium, manganese, magnesium, sodium and iron, flavonoids, saponins, tannins, vitamins B1, B2, B3 and C, bitter substances, organic acids, essential oils, traces of alkaloids.

## Use
Fresh, green, mature spikes (the harder they feel, the more silicon they contain).

# NETTLE RINSE FOR SKIN AND HAIR

This rinse will strengthen your scalp as well as your hair and is also effective for oily scalps. You can also add rosemary to boost the circulation in your scalp, or greater burdock to strengthen the roots of your hair and combat hair loss.

**Ingredients for 500ml**
• Approx. 100g (one handful) nettle tips
• 500ml boiling water

Pick the nettle tips and pour the boiling water over them. Leave to infuse for ten minutes then allow to cool before applying to your hair and scalp. You can also drink the nettle water to strengthen your hair from the inside out.

# FIELD HORSETAIL INFUSION

Field horsetail is rich in silicon, although you need to boil it for a short period to release the mineral. The decoction will strengthen your hair, nails and bones.

**Ingredients for 500ml**
• Approx. 100g (one handful) field horsetail
• 500ml water

Place the field horsetail and water in a pan, boil for 20 minutes and leave to cool. Strain and apply to your hair, leaving it to penetrate before you rinse it off.

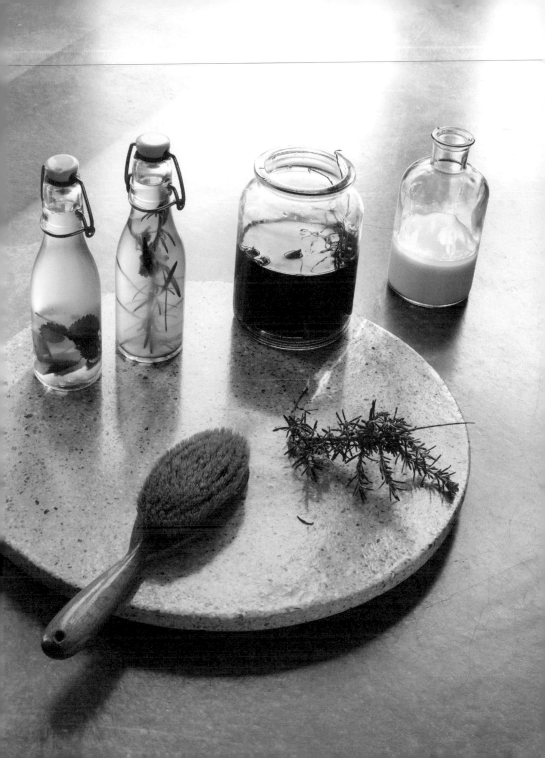

# MASKS FOR YOUR HAIR

When you apply a hair mask (also known as a deep conditioning treatment), always leave it for a while so that the active ingredients can penetrate deep into your hair.

## WARM OIL MASK WITH CAMOMILE

Infusing camomile in oil is a good way to make an oil mask for dry hair.

**Ingredients for 1 mask**
- 50ml olive oil
- 10g camomile flowers
- 5 drops neem oil

Heat the olive oil and camomile flowers in a water bath, leaving them to infuse for at least 20 minutes (the longer you leave them, the better). Add the neem oil, strain to remove the camomile flowers and apply the oil to your hair while it is still warm. Wrap your hair in aluminium foil to allow the mask to penetrate properly, leave for half an hour and then wash out with shampoo.

## RICE WATER

The water that you strain off after cooking rice is nourishing for your hair. Simply apply, leave for half an hour to penetrate and then wash out. Rice water is also an effective spray for curly hair, as is oatmeal water.

## COCONUT MILK

When it comes to beauty products, there's more to coconuts than just the oil; coconut milk is also nourishing for your hair and scalp. Take a tin of coconut milk, heat the contents to body temperature and apply to your hair. Leave for half an hour to penetrate and then wash out with shampoo.

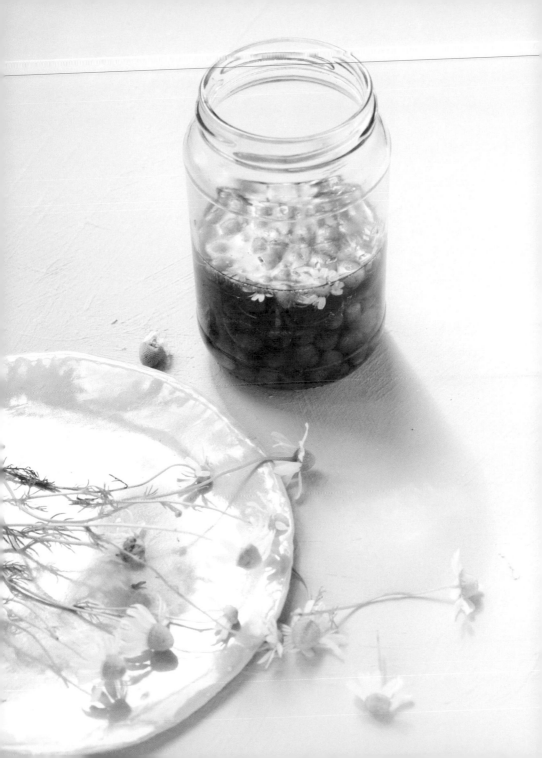

# ROSEMARY COCONUT OIL

Rosemary boosts the circulation in your scalp, while coconut provides excellent nourishment for your hair and scalp.

## Ingredients for 100ml
- 100g coconut oil
- 5 stems fresh rosemary with leaves and any flowers
- A clean 100ml pot or jar

Heat the coconut oil and rosemary stems, turn the heat down low and leave to infuse for half an hour. Remove from the heat and leave for another 24 hours to infuse and cool. Reheat and strain the oil into the pot, leaving it to cool and set slightly. Apply as a mask, leave for half an hour to penetrate and then wash out with shampoo.

# ROSEMARY HAIR WATER

If you don't want to apply anything oily to your scalp but you do want to benefit from the properties of rosemary, you can also use the herb to make a powerful decoction. Heat the stems of rosemary with half a litre of water and turn the heat down low as soon as it comes to the boil. Leave to infuse for 20 minutes over a low heat, then remove from the heat, strain and leave to cool. Apply to your scalp and leave to penetrate for half an hour, then rinse your hair to remove.

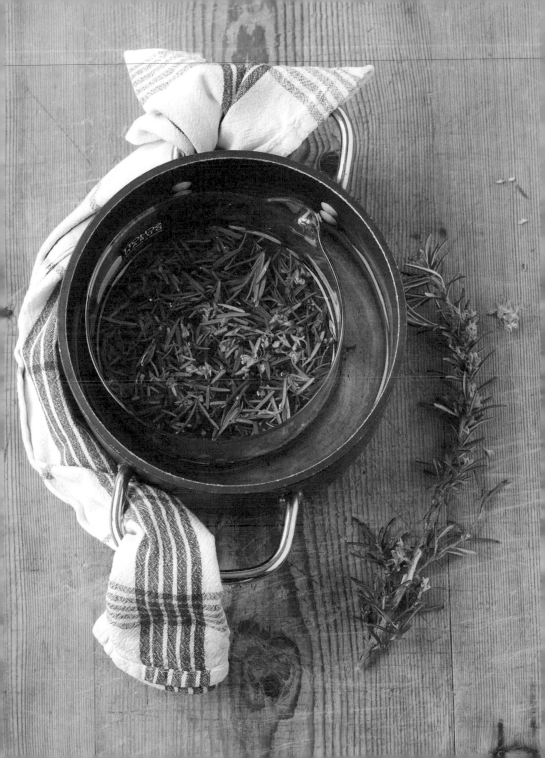

# HAIR-CARE BOOSTERS

## ROSEMARY WAX

This wax is wonderfully nourishing and nurturing for dry and split ends.

### Ingredients for 120g
- 100ml infused rosemary oil (see pages 12-13 for how to make a macerated oil)
- 20g beeswax
- Six small 20g pots with lids

Heat the beeswax in a water bath until it melts. Add the rosemary oil and mix thoroughly. Transfer to the pots and leave to set. Before applying the wax to your hair, rub it between your palms to warm and soften it.

## LINSEED GEL

Scrunching linseed gel into your hair is an excellent way to make sure that your curls are sleek and defined.

### Ingredients for 100ml
- 20g (2 tbsp) linseeds
- 100ml water
- A sieve (not too fine)
- A clean 100ml pot or jar with lid

Mix the linseeds and water, leave overnight and the next day you will have a gel-like substance. Strain the linseeds out of the gel, which is then ready for use. Store the remaining gel in the jar or pot with the lid on.

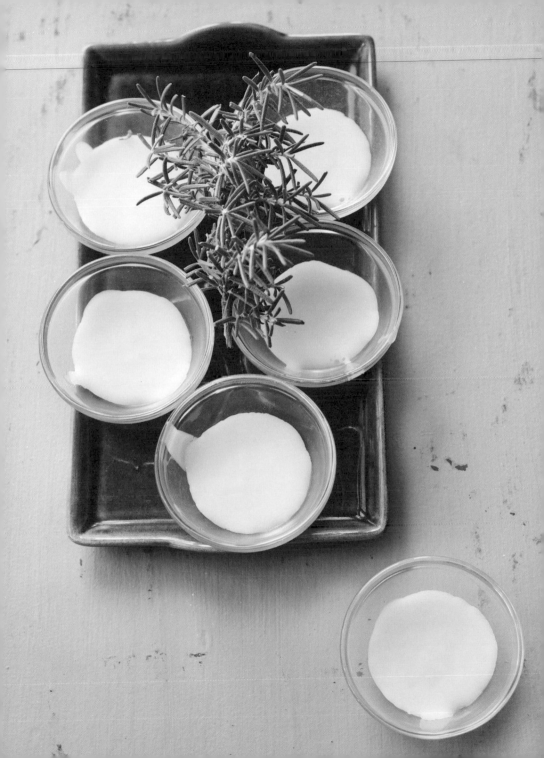

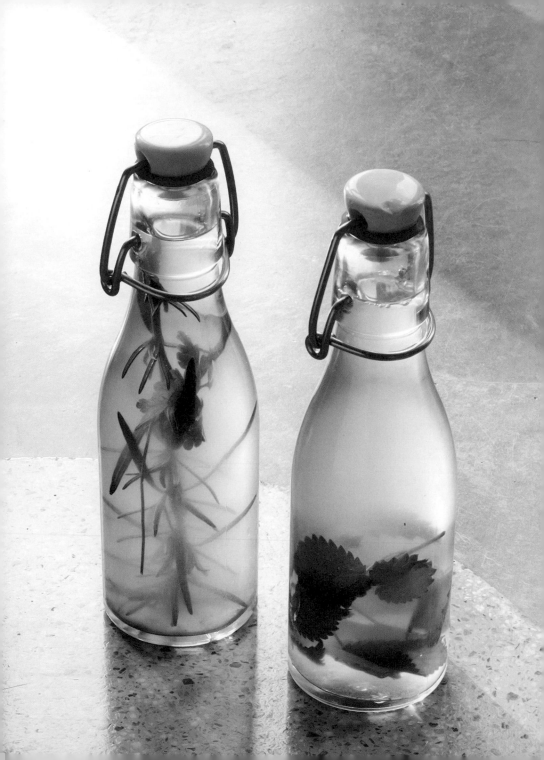

# HAIR SERUM

This serum is another excellent way to stop the ends of your hair from drying out.

**Ingredients for 30ml**
- 15ml argan oil
- 15ml sesame oil
- 10 drops vitamin E oil
- 10 drops camomile oil or another infused oil of your choice
- A clean 30ml bottle with cap

Mix the oils thoroughly and transfer to the bottle. Apply the mixture to the ends of your hair as a serum.

# HAIR MIST

This mist is an effective treatment for dry and damaged hair.

**Ingredients for 50ml**
- 40ml rosewater or another hydrolate of your choice
- 30ml aloe vera gel
- 5ml (1 tsp) organic honey
- 5ml glycerin
- A clean 50ml spray bottle

Place the aloe vera gel and rosewater in a pan and heat gently. Add the honey and allow to melt, then add the glycerin and mix thoroughly. Leave the mixture to cool and decant into the spray bottle.

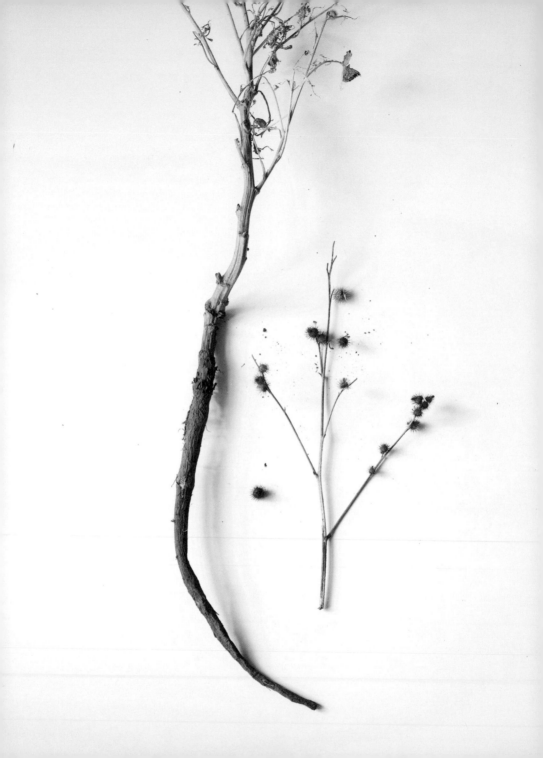

# GREATER BURDOCK
(Arctium lappa)

Asteraceae

Greater burdock is effective against skin problems like eczema and fungal infections, plus it helps to prevent hair loss.

## Effect on the skin and hair
Antibacterial (including against staphylococci and streptococci) and antifungal.

## When to use
For hair loss, dandruff and an oily scalp. On your skin: for sores, abscesses, boils, fungal infections, erysipelas, acne, eczema and other flaking skin conditions.

## Active ingredients
Carbohydrates, phenolic acids, bitter substances, phytosterols, greasy oil, organic acids, flavonol glycosides, minerals including potassium, calcium, magnesium and iron, and vitamins including B1, B2, B3, B6, B12, C and E.

## Use
The dried root of a plant in its second year (harvested in the summer or autumn) for a tincture, decoction or extract. The leaves are sometimes used to make macerations in olive oil to treat leg ulcers. They can also be pounded to make a poultice.

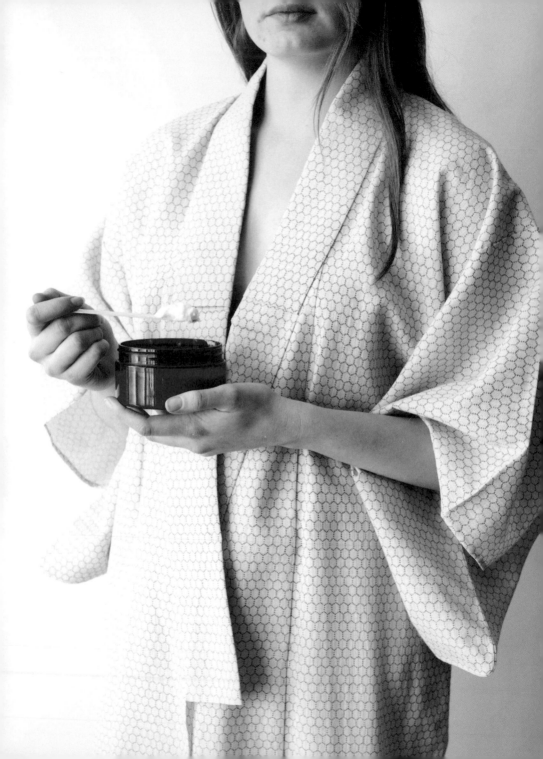

# LOOKING AFTER YOUR BODY

Make a lovely nigella oil and use it to look after your body or treat yourself all over with a flower bath. Use sage powder on your feet and soak your hands with camomile.

## NIGELLA OIL

Morocco and neighbouring countries primarily use nigella seed to make face and body oil that combats premature aging and fortifies your skin. You can also use the oil to cleanse skin imperfections. Nigella seed is available from a variety of outlets, including Moroccan shops. If you cannot find any, you can replace it with cumin seed.

**Ingredients for 100ml**
- 100ml oil such as almond or argan oil
- 20g nigella seed
- A pestle and mortar
- A clean 100ml pot or jar with lid
- Muslin

Grind the seeds slightly in the pestle and mortar and place them in the pot. Pour over the oil to slightly below the top of the pot. Cover with muslin (not the lid) and leave to stand for four weeks, stirring occasionally. Strain the oil after four weeks and store in the clean pot with the lid on.

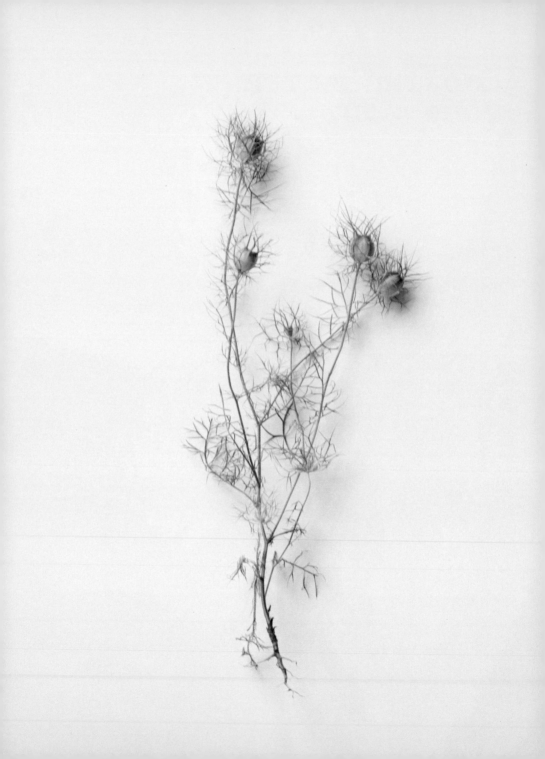

# LOVE-IN-A-MIST WITH BLACK CUMIN SEED

(Nigella damascena and Nigella sativa)

Ranunculaceae

Both types of nigella seed and the oil from them have long been taken as medicine to boost the immune system and treat allergies, asthma and bronchitis. Women in Ancient Egypt also ate the seeds to make their breasts firmer and more toned. The seeds are often used to produce oil: black seed oil or black cumin oil.

## Effect on the skin
Strengthening, hydrating and cleansing.

## When to use
For premature skin aging, eczema, psoriasis and acne.

## Active ingredients
Fatty acids, bioflavonoids, phytonutrients, amino acids, proteins, omega 3, 6 and 9 fatty acids.

## Use
The seeds for a cold-pressed or infused oil.

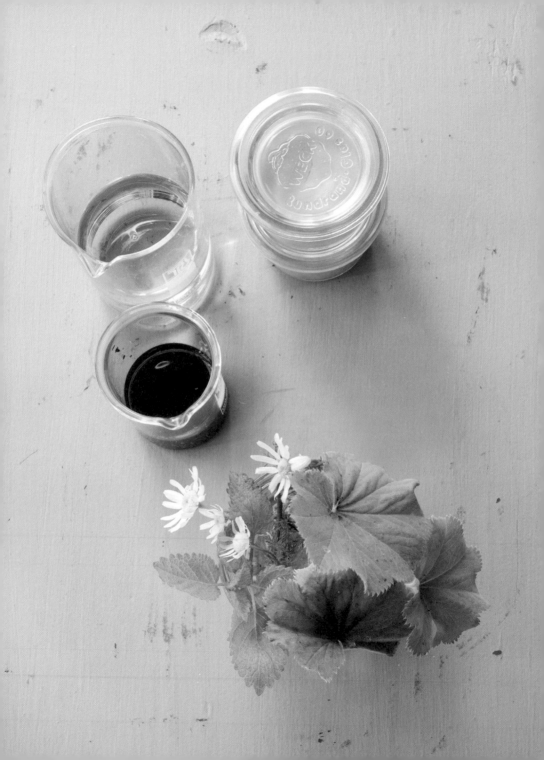

# CREAM FOR YOUR NECK, CHEST AND BREASTS

This cream containing nigella, lady's mantle and camomile is wonderful for your neck, chest and breasts, but you can also tweak the ingredients and use other plants such as marjoram and yarrow.

Make nigella oil (see page 143) and St John's oil (see page 71). You will also need a camomile and lady's mantle infusion (see page 183) with 50-100g flowers and 150ml boiled water, as well as a lady's mantle tincture (see pages 10-11 for how to make a tincture) with 50-100g flowers and 175ml vodka.

## Ingredients for 250ml
- 10g beeswax
- 20ml nigella oil
- 20ml St John's oil (this will colour the cream a beautiful pink)
- 20g emulsifier
- 100ml camomile and lady's mantle infusion
- 50ml lady's mantle tincture
- 50ml aloe vera gel
- A clean 250ml pot or jar with lid

## Optional
- 20 drops essential oil in a blend of your choice
- 5 drops vitamin E oil
- 1 tbsp witch hazel hydrolate (see page 31)

Melt the beeswax in a water bath, then add the oils and emulsifier. Place the camomile and lady's mantle infusion, lady's mantle tincture and aloe vera gel in a different small pan and heat. Make sure that both mixtures are at approximately the same temperature, then slowly combine them, stirring continuously until they are thoroughly blended and you have a smooth, homogenous cream. Add the essential oil, vitamin E oil and witch hazel hydrolate (if you are using them) and mix thoroughly again. Transfer to the pot, leave to cool and then put the lid on the pot and add a label.

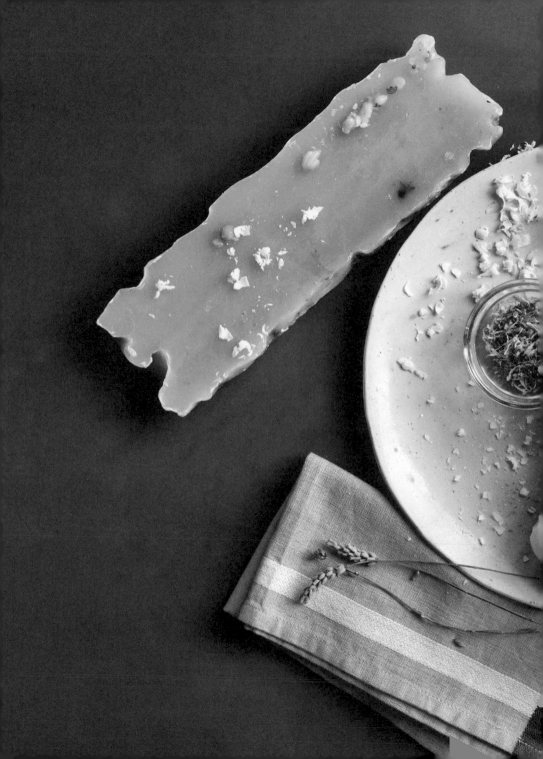

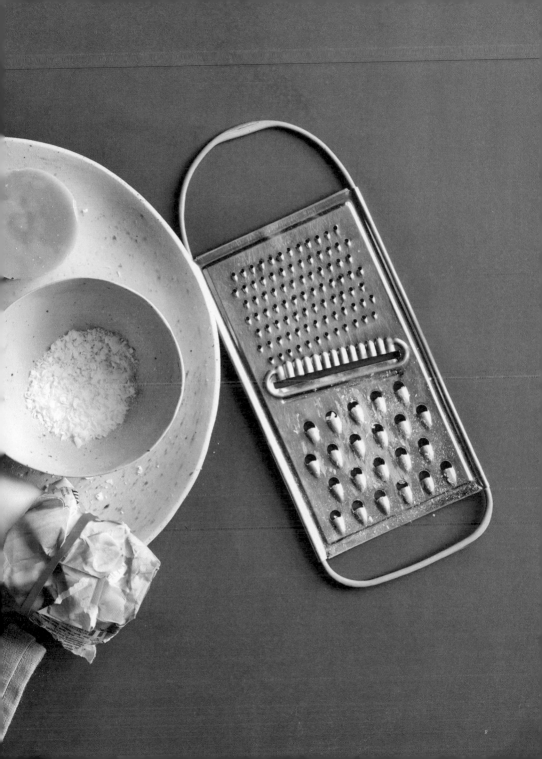

# HERB ROBERT
## (Geranium robertianum)

Geraniaceae

Herb Robert has a blood-red stem that looks a bit like a vein, which is how I remember that this plant is good for blood vessels. Applied externally to soothe bruises and contusions; do not use if pregnant or breastfeeding.

## When to use
For contusions, bruises and minor cuts.

## Active ingredients
Tannins, bitter substances, organic acids, essential oil, resin, gum, pectin, vitamin C.

## Use
The whole plant, including the root. Used to make a compress.

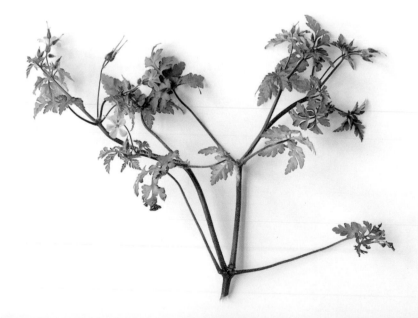

# RINSE AND COMPRESS USING HERB ROBERT

**Ingredients for 500ml**
- 50g herb Robert
- 500ml water
- A clean heat-proof 750ml bottle or jug

Place the herb Robert in the bottle and add a dash of cold water. Bring the remaining water to the boil, remove from the heat and immediately pour it over the herb Robert. Leave to cool until it reaches body temperature. Use to flush out cuts and wounds, or to make a compress.

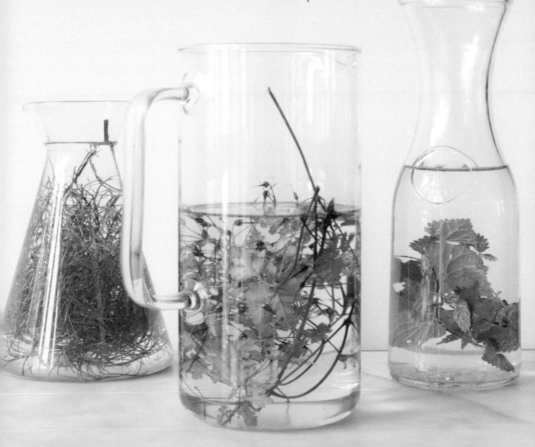

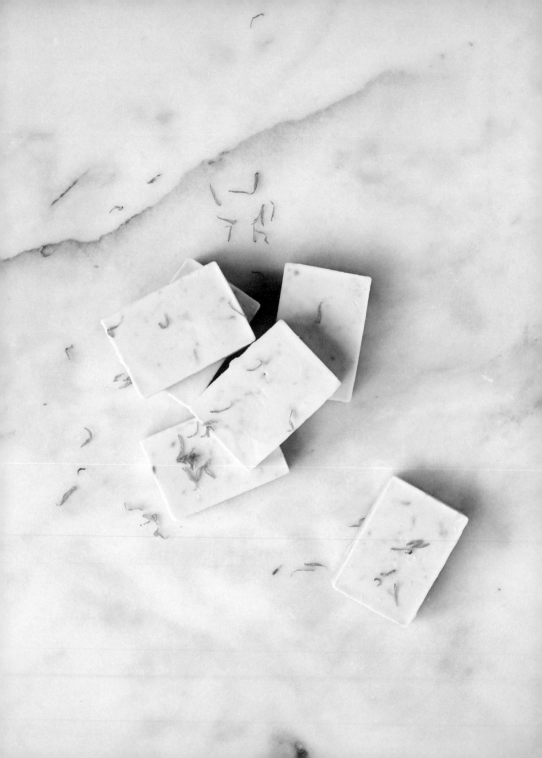

# MARLIES VAN HEUSDEN'S MARIGOLD SOAP

Marlies van Heusden from Nature Bar has a workshop in Amsterdam where she makes soap from wonderful ingredients, including marigold, lavender, mint and shea butter. But with the circular economy in mind, she also incorporates waste products like used coffee from the café on the corner (the residual caffeine is great for skin and coffee grounds make an excellent scrub), orange peel from the juice machine in the local supermarket (they smell wonderful) and rose petals from roses rejected by the local florist (rose is astringent, nourishing and has an amazing fragrance).

Although her time in Mexico inspired Marlies to start making soap, she's been aware of the power of marigold (calendula) since she was a child, when marigold ointment was her mother's universal remedy. If Marlies cut herself, her mother would apply marigold ointment. If she was in pain or had an itch, she turned to marigold ointment. When Marlies was in Mexico, she struggled with mosquito bites that itched so much that she scratched them until they bled. She couldn't get hold of any marigold ointment but she did find marigold soap which was very effective, restorative and healing for her mosquito bites. Inspired by the fact that soap could be made with marigold, she realized that a whole host of other ingredients could also be used. And that's what she did. Read on for Marlies's account of how to make soap.

Marlies: 'I use the cold-process method to make soaps and shampoo bars by hand for Nature Bar, my business. This artisan method is the purest and most authentic way of making soap.

'Although it takes quite a long time for the soap to cure completely – between four and six weeks – your patience will be rewarded! The low processing temperatures not only ensure that as many of the vitamins and minerals as possible are retained but also enhance and optimize the positive qualities of the soap's ingredients.

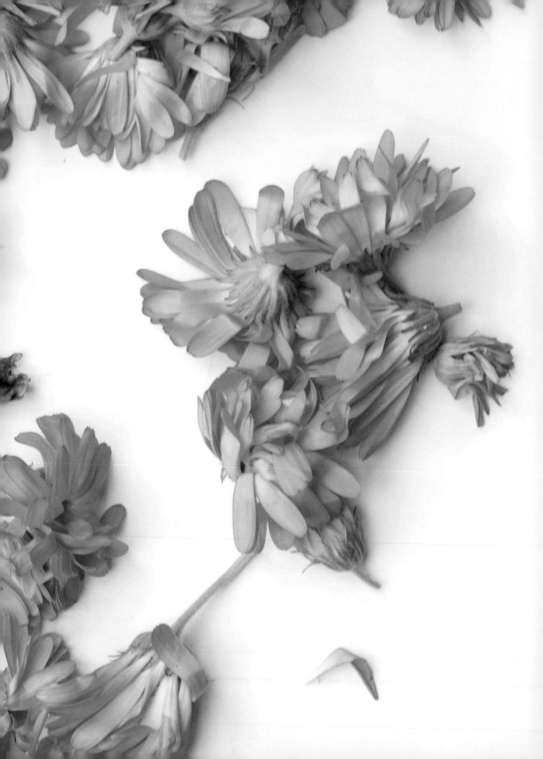

'These days, practically all soap is made by machines using the hot-process method, generally because it is faster and much cheaper than making artisan, handmade soap using the cold-process method. Not only does the high temperature destroy many of the minerals and vitamins, but manufacturers often also choose the cheapest ingredients, ignoring the environmental impact of using them.

'Comparing factory-produced soap with handmade, cold-process soap is a bit like comparing factory-produced bread with sourdough bread from an artisan baker.

'You only need three basic ingredients for the cold-process method: a fat, water and sodium hydroxide – although you can also add fragrances and pigments. I choose to make pure, natural soap and I only add natural ingredients like essential oils and different types of clay.

'The chemical reaction between the fat and water with sodium hydroxide (which combine to form lye) triggers the saponification process that ultimately produces handmade soap. Once the saponification process is complete and the soap is fully cured, no trace of the lye remains.

'Making soap is a magical process and every time is different from the one before. It might seem simple because there are so few ingredients, but it really is all about the interplay between the ingredients, the temperatures and how long you spend mixing. The end result is a mild, luxurious soap that cleanses and nourishes your skin.

'My products are unique because each soap and shampoo bar contains a circular ingredient; in other words, a product that is being reused, like coffee grounds or orange peel. As my Orange & Marigold soap is a real crowd pleaser, I've added a simplified version to this basic recipe as an extra treat so you can also make circular soap and help to create a cleaner and more beautiful world.

'The recipe that I'm sharing with you here is for the very first soap I ever made. It's also the recipe that led me to fall in love with making soap.'

## Equipment
- Safety glasses & gloves
- Face mask
- Two glass measuring jugs for the lye mixture
- Weighing scales
- Spoon
- Thermometer

- Additional measuring jug
- Pan
- Fine grater
- Soap mould; an empty milk carton, for example, or a (silicone) baking tin
- Old tea towel or hand towel
- Sieve
- Whisk (or alternatively a hand blender)
- Spatula

## Ingredients

### Lye mixture
- 149g water (weigh it out into a dish on the weighing scales)
- 65g lye crystals

### Base oils
- 150g olive oil
- 150g coconut oil
- 150g sunflower oil (infused with marigold)

### Additional ingredients
- 15g orange oil
- 1 tsp grated orange peel
- 5g marigold petals (dried)

## Step 1
### Lye mixture
Lye needs to be handled with care, so put on the gloves and wear the safety glasses and face mask. Put the water in one glass measuring jug and the lye crystals (sodium hydroxide) in the other. Working in a well-ventilated space – below the extractor hood, for example, or outdoors – add the lye crystals to the water. Never pour the water onto the lye crystals! Immediately stir the crystals carefully with a spoon until they have dissolved fully into the water. The crystals release a lot of heat as they dissolve so make sure that the measuring jug is in a safe spot where the lye mixture can cool until it is 40-50°C and transparent.

## Step 2
### Base oils
Weigh out the oils and place them in the pan. Put the pan on a low heat until the coconut oil melts and forms an emulsion with the other oils. Monitor the temperature carefully and do not allow the oils to become hotter than 45°C, as this will destroy their positive qualities.

## Step 3
### Additional ingredients
Weigh out the orange oil, grated orange peel and marigold petals and place them in the second measuring jug. I use the peel from oranges juiced in a local supermarket but you can also grate the peel of a fresh orange.

## Step 4
### Final preparations
Put your mould out ready on a tea towel or hand towel. Check your

temperatures. Once both the oils and the lye mixture are at around 45°C, you can start the most enjoyable step of the process.

## Step 5
### Making soap
Now it's time to start making your soap. To start the saponification process, carefully pour the lye mixture through the sieve into the oil mixture. Almost immediately, you'll see the transparent, golden oil mixture transform into a cloudier mixture that is lighter in colour. Use the whisk to gently stir the mixture in the pan until it thickens to the consistency of custard – this may take a while. Although you can use a hand blender instead of the whisk if you're in a hurry, as this will really speed up the saponification process, I would advise novice soap makers to be patient and use the whisk.

You can check whether your mixture has reached the correct consistency by testing for trace, which means that it is thick enough to leave a trail on the surface. Dip the whisk into the soap mixture and let a few drips fall onto the surface of the mixture. If they remain visible – even if only briefly – then it's thick enough.

Add the orange oil, grated orange peel and marigold petals, stirring again with the whisk until they are completely incorporated into the soap mixture. Pour the soap into the mould, using the spatula to scrape the pan completely empty. Tap the mould carefully on the counter to distribute the soap mixture evenly, then cover it with the tea towel or hand towel and leave the mixture so the saponification process can continue.

Make sure that you remember to keep your gloves on while you are cleaning up. The lye mixture in fresh soap is not completely dissolved, so you don't want it to come into contact with your skin!

Leave the soap in the mould for a day or two, then remove it and cut into bars of the size you want. Put them in a dry place to cure for four to six weeks, then they are ready for use.

'Let's raise the bar together!'

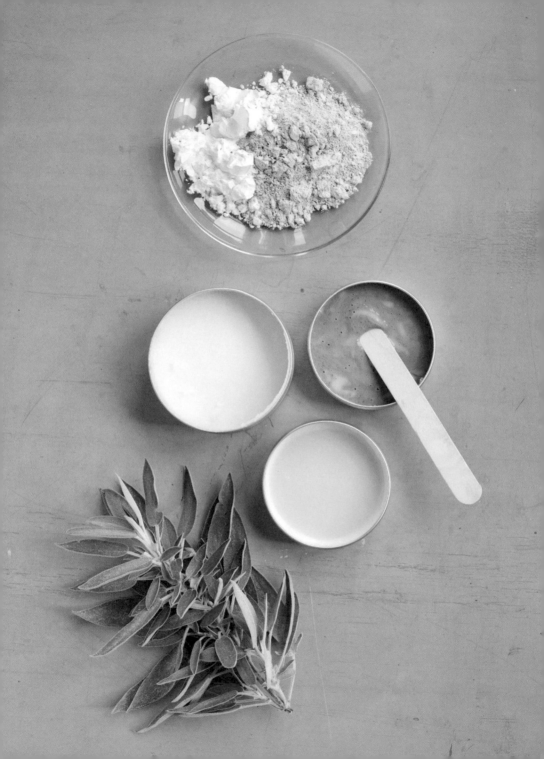

# DEODORANTS

Shop-bought deodorants tend to be full of substances that aren't great for your skin, including strong fragrances and aluminium, but making your own is very easy. If you choose that option, I recommend taking the time to decide which recipe will work best for you.

## CREAM DEODORANT WITH BAKING SODA

Baking soda is a common ingredient in deodorants.

### Ingredients for approximately 100g

- 40g coconut oil
- 40g cornflour
- 8g baking soda
- 20 drops essential oil, such as lavender, sage or pine
- A clean 100g pot or jar with lid

Mix the coconut oil and cornflour. Add the baking soda, mixing thoroughly, followed by the essential oil. Keep in the pot with the lid on.

## CREAM DEODORANT WITH ARROWROOT

Some people's skin reacts poorly to baking soda. If you are one of them, you can use arrowroot powder instead, or give this recipe a try:

### Ingredients for approximately 100g

- 50g beeswax
- 30ml infused oil from a plant of your choice
- 25g shea butter
- 20 drops essential oil of your choice
- 20g (4 tbsp) arrowroot powder
- A clean 100g aluminium pot or jar with lid

Melt the beeswax in a water bath, then add the infused oil and mix with the wax. Add the shea butter and leave to melt, then remove from the heat and add the essential oil. Finally, add the arrowroot powder and mix thoroughly. Transfer to the pot and put the lid on.

# COMMON SAGE
(Salvia officinalis)

Lamiaceae

'Sage' is taken from the Latin 'salvare', which means to heal, rescue, redeem or sanctify. In the past, the herb was deemed to be holy and was a common remedy. Sage is rich in antioxidants.

## Effect on the skin
Antiperspirant.

## When to use
For excessive perspiration, sweaty palms, sweaty feet and night sweats.

## Active ingredients
Essential oil (including thujone, eucalyptol, borneol and camphor), tannins, bitter substances, saponins, organic acids, minerals including sodium, potassium, calcium, iron and silicon, B vitamins, gum and resin.

## Use
The fresh leaves before the plant flowers.

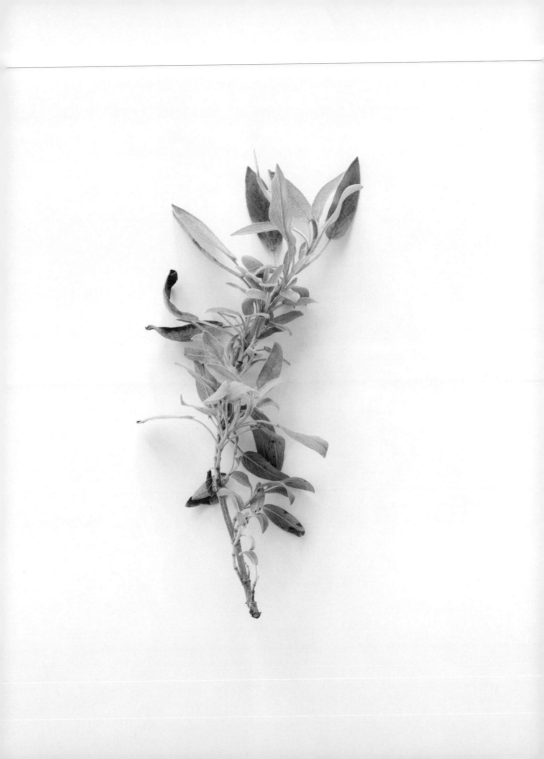

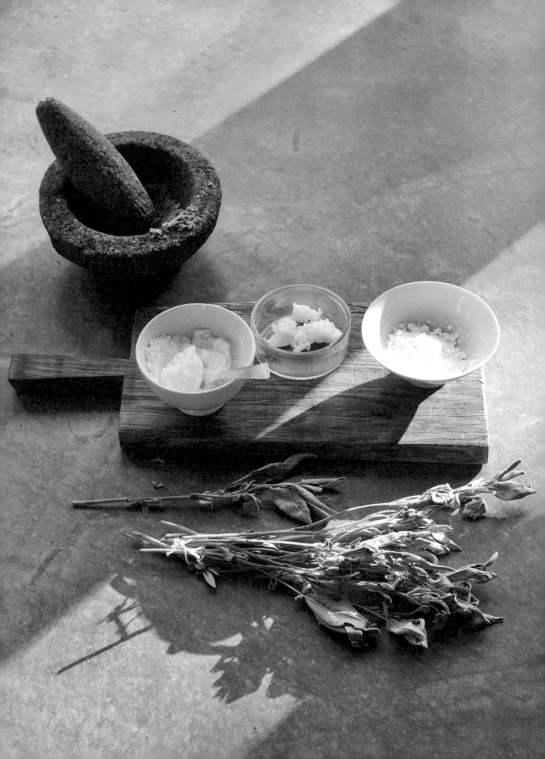

# CREAM DEODORANT WITH WHITE CLAY

The mixture will set quickly as it cools, making it harder to combine the ingredients thoroughly, so make sure you have all your ingredients and equipment to hand so that you can work quickly. If the mixture still becomes too hard before it is thoroughly mixed, simply melt it again and continue.

**Ingredients for approximately 100g**
- 10g cocoa butter
- 40g shea butter
- 15g beeswax
- 30g kaolin white clay (powder)
- 7 drops essential lavender oil
- 7 drops essential tea tree oil
- A clean 100g pot or jar with lid

Melt the cocoa butter slowly over a low heat. Add the shea butter and beeswax and allow them to melt. Remove from the heat, add the clay and mix. Finally, add the essential oils and mix everything thoroughly. Transfer to the pot and put the lid on.

# POWDER DEODORANT

Use this recipe if you prefer a dry powder deodorant.

**Ingredients for approximately 100g**
- 5 stems dried sage
- 40g cornflour
- 40g kaolin white or green clay (powder)
- 5g baking soda
- 20 drops essential oil (pine, tea tree or eucalyptus)
- Pestle and mortar
- Shaker

Place the dried sage in the pestle and mortar and grind to a powder. Place the cornflour, clay and baking soda in a bowl, then add the sage and essential oil. Mix thoroughly to form a fine powder, then transfer to the shaker.

# BATHING, SHOWERING AND SCRUBBING

## Flower baths

A flower bath is an opportunity not only to enjoy a wonderful fragrance, but also to adjust how energetic you feel. Depending on the flowers you choose, it can be stimulating or calming, reinvigorating or nourishing. I'd need a whole book to explain the effects of all the different flowers, so here are just a few:

- Rose petals have an astringent effect on the skin and encourage us to look after ourselves.
- Lavender flowers help you wind down and relax at bedtime and have an antibacterial effect on your bladder and urinary tract. They help you to balance your emotions and boost your self-acceptance and self-confidence. Lavender is also effective for anxiety about aging.
- Camomile flowers are soothing and calming, as well as boosting your self-acceptance and self-confidence.
- Arnica flowers warm your muscles and promote calm, as well as boosting your self-confidence.

### TIP
You can either use the flowers or add a few drops of essential oil to your bath oil or bathwater. You can also make a maceration (see pages 12–13).

## SWEET BODY SCRUB

My 11-year-old daughter, Juna, often uses sugar for a wonderful body scrub that's super simple to make. If you think that sugar isn't that good for your skin, you couldn't be more wrong; both sugar and honey have excellent healing properties. Hospitals will sometimes use sugar or honey to treat pressure sores with outstanding results.

### Ingredients for 75ml
- 60g (2 tsp) organic cane sugar
- 30ml olive oil (or a plant-infused oil)
- 30ml runny organic honey
- 5 drops essential oil of your choice
- A clean 75ml pot with lid

Mix the ingredients thoroughly and transfer them to the pot.

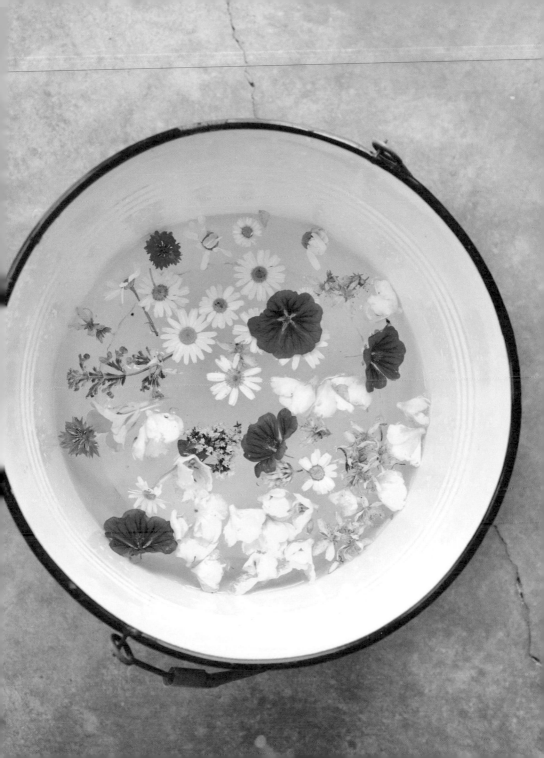

# BATH BOMB WITH LAVENDER

You can buy bath bomb moulds online so making bath bombs is child's play.

## Ingredients for 1 bath bomb (150g)

- 1½g dried lavender
- 90g baking soda
- 45g citric acid
- 12g cornflour
- 10 drops essential lavender oil
- A few drops of water or hydrolate of your choice
- Pestle and mortar

Place the lavender in the pestle and mortar and grind to a powder. Mix all the dry ingredients in a dish or bowl. Add the essential oil and mix thoroughly. Add a few drops of water or hydrolate and mix again until it feels like wet sand. Transfer to the two halves of the mould, filling one half slightly more than the other so they will combine properly to form a whole. Press the two halves of the mould together with a twisting motion, then remove the bath bomb and leave for two hours to dry.

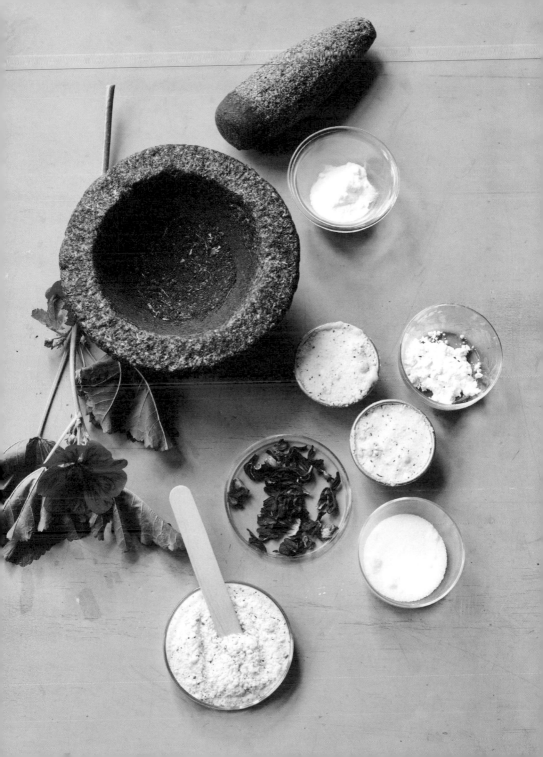

# AYURVEDIC SHOWER GEL

You only need a few ingredients to make yourself a wonderful shower gel. This recipe comes from ayurveda; a traditional medicine system that is based on three different categories – vata, pitta and kapha. It can be interesting to find out what category you fall into and what foods and ingredients you should both prioritize and avoid. For the sake of convenience, however, this recipe is based on the following principles: use sesame oil for dry skin (vata), coconut oil for sensitive skin (pitta) and sunflower oil for oily skin (kapha). You can tweak these principles and adapt the recipe to suit your own understanding by blending or adding oils.

### Ingredients for 150ml
• 60ml Castile soap
• 60ml coconut, sesame or sunflower oil
• 30ml runny organic honey
• A clean 150ml pump bottle

Place the ingredients in a bowl and mix thoroughly, then transfer to the pump bottle. Shake well before use.

# BATH SALTS WITH MARJORAM

Adding herbs to your bath salts is very easy; simply grind them finely first in the pestle and mortar. Marjoram calms the nervous system and is therefore a wonderful choice, or you can opt for lavender or sage.

### Ingredients for 1 bath
• 5 stems dried marjoram
• 150g Dead Sea salt
• Pestle and mortar

Dry the marjoram stems, then strip off the leaves and flowers and grind them to powder in the pestle and mortar. Add the salt to the powder and mix.

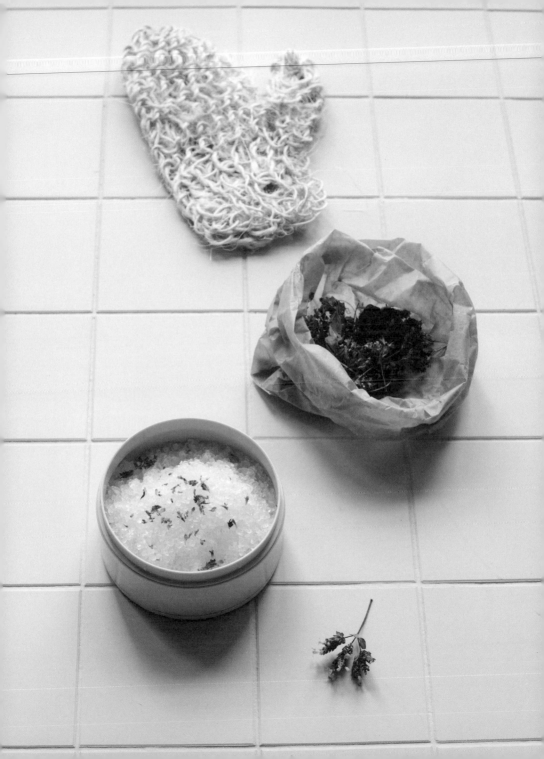

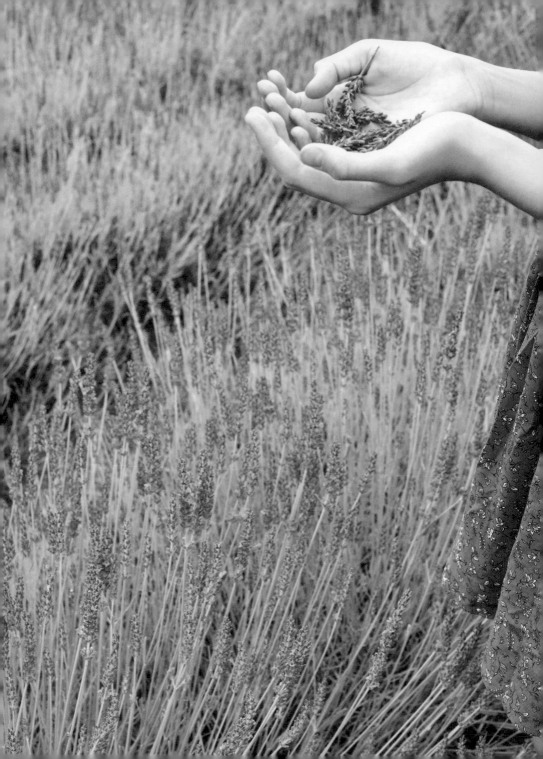

# LAVENDER
## (Lavandula angustifolia)

Lamiaceae

Essential lavender oil is often used because of its
antibacterial, antiviral and antifungal effects, while the
wonderful fragrance calms your nervous system and promotes
good sleep.

## Effect on the skin
Disinfectant, antibacterial, antiviral and antifungal.
Analgesic and repels insects.
Lavender also has the following effect on your nervous
system: calming, relaxing, balancing and promotes sleep.

## When to use
For relatively minor first-degree burns, sunburn, (infected)
wounds, insect bites, cold sores and head lice, as well as
for anxiety, stress, restlessness and sleep issues.

## Active ingredients
Essential oil, tannins, bitter substances, triterpenes,
phenolic acids and flavonoids.

## Use
The flowers for a tincture, infusion or tea.
Essential oil: 1 to 3 drops essential oil to 1 tablespoon
of carrier oil.
You can also use decoctions and finely ground powder, or
make lavender ointment, vinegar, oil or honey.

## SKIN OIL WITH LAVENDER

The perfect time to apply a luxurious oil is when your skin is still damp and warm from your bath – your skin will absorb it better so you won't need to use as much.

**Ingredients for 100ml**
- 10g lavender flowers
- 100ml almond oil or another oil of your choice
- A clean 100ml pot or jar
- A clean 100ml bottle with cap

Fill the pot with the lavender flowers and pour over the oil to cover them. Cover the pot with a cotton cloth and leave to stand for six weeks, stirring occasionally.

Shortcut: heat the oil with the lavender in a water bath for around 48 hours. Stir occasionally and make sure that there is always water in the bath. Turn the heat off at night and on again the next morning, so you can monitor it consistently.

For both versions, finish by straining the oil and pouring it into the bottle.

## BODY BUTTER WITH LAVENDER

This body butter contains lavender and is a little thicker in consistency. The perfect time to apply it is in the evening, as lavender will calm your mind and promote a good night's sleep. You can use a different essential oil instead if you prefer.

**Ingredients for approximately 150ml**
- 50g coconut oil
- 100g shea butter
- 10ml (1 tbsp) infused camomile oil
- 20 drops essential lavender oil
- A clean 150ml pot or jar with lid

Heat the coconut oil until it melts. Place the shea butter in a separate bowl and beat until it is soft and creamy. Pour the melted coconut oil onto the shea butter, add the camomile oil and mix together. Finally, add the lavender oil and mix again. Transfer the body butter to the pot and put the lid on.

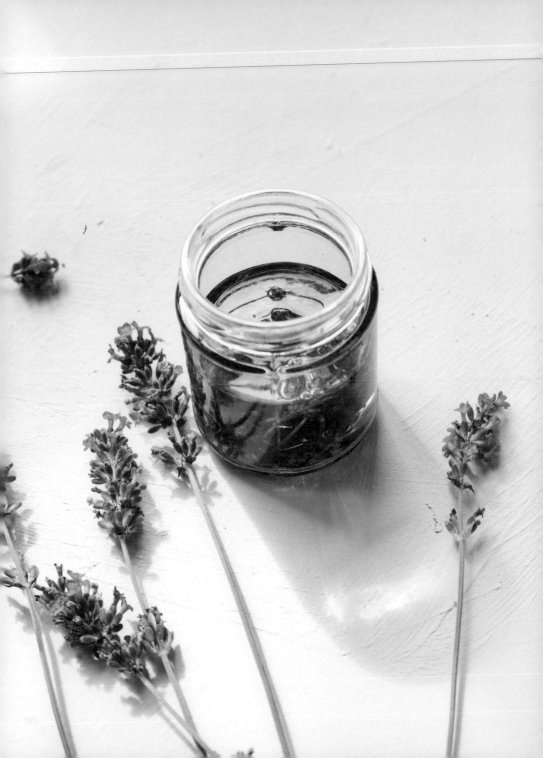

# BODY MILK WITH ROSEMARY OR LAVENDER

Essential rosemary oil stimulates your nervous system. Centuries ago, the oil was used by Romans, Greeks and Egyptians, who regarded it as holy. Rosemary oil stimulates your circulation, eases headaches and nerve pain, and activates your whole system, so it's the perfect choice for a body milk that you apply in the morning.

**Ingredients for approximately 200ml**
- 100g shea butter
- 100g coconut oil
- 10ml (1 tbsp) infused camomile oil
- 10ml (1 tbsp) argan oil
- 20 drops essential rosemary or lavender oil
- Hand blender
- A clean 200ml pot or jar with lid

Heat the shea butter briefly until it melts. Add the coconut oil and mix with the hand blender until it is light and fluffy. Add the camomile and argan oils, followed by the essential rosemary oil. Mix thoroughly and transfer to the pot.

# BABY OINTMENT WITH ZINC TO PREVENT NAPPY RASH

Nappy rash can be really distressing for your baby, so this gentle baby ointment is perfect.

**Ingredients for approximately 185g**
- 125g coconut oil
- 2g (1 tbsp) marigold flowers
- 2g (1 tbsp) camomile flowers
- 60g shea butter
- 5g (1 tsp) zinc oxide (powder)
- Muslin
- A clean 185g pot or jar with lid

Place the coconut oil in a small bowl and melt in a water bath. Add the marigold and chamomile flowers and leave to infuse for a couple of hours, making sure that the water does not evaporate completely. Once the coconut oil has turned a golden colour and has a wonderful fragrance of the flowers in it, strain it through muslin. Add the shea butter and mix (melt it briefly first, if necessary, to make this easier). Add the zinc oxide, mix thoroughly and pour into the pot.

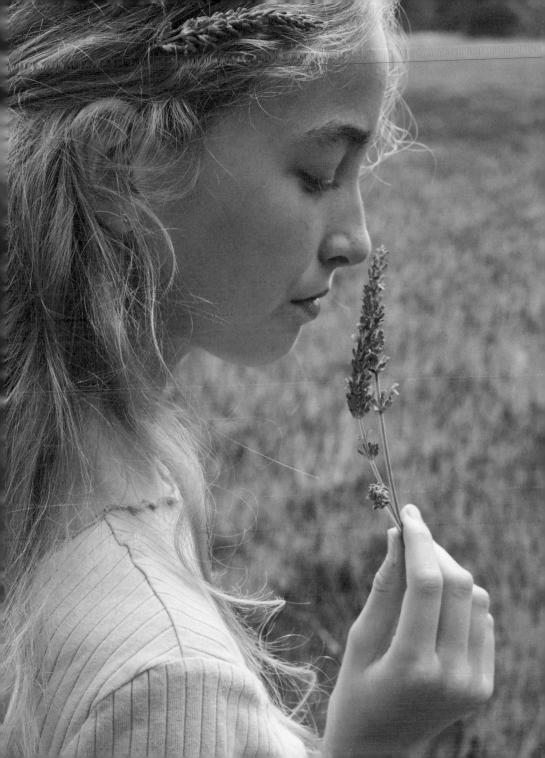

# GINGER
## (Zingiber officinale)

Zingiberaceae

Although ginger has become a staple ingredient in the West, the root (technically a rhizome) is native to India and is now cultivated in Southeast Asia, as well as many other tropical and subtropical countries. Ginger is commonly used in ayurvedic and Chinese cuisine.

## Effect on the skin
Anti-inflammatory and analgesic. Boosts your circulation and thus the blood supply to your skin.

## When to use
For blemished skin and acne, minor wounds and poor circulation (chilblains and numb hands and feet).

## Active ingredients
Essential oil, oleoresins, phenols, enzymes, vitamins B1, B2, B3, B6, C and beta-carotene, minerals including calcium, magnesium, phosphorus, potassium and selenium, wax, carbohydrates, proteins, organic acids and fibre.

## Use
The roots (ideally the smaller, young ones).

# GINGER OIL

Ginger is a delicious ingredient in Easter dishes or golden milk (almond milk with turmeric and cinnamon). It is also an excellent ingredient in skin care products. Ginger oil is easy to make, has a wonderful fragrance and is good for your circulation. It is effective against inflammation of your joints and skin, plus it eases muscle pain, so don't forget to apply it after training.

### Ingredients for 100ml
- 10g ginger root
- 100ml almond oil
- A clean 100ml pot or jar
- A clean 100ml bottle with cap

Slice the ginger root into rounds and place them in the pot. Add the oil and heat in a water bath. Leave to infuse for around half an hour, then strain the oil. Pour it into the bottle and close with the cap.

# ARNICA
(Arnica montana)

Asteraceae

Arnica has beautiful yellow flowers and is most often found in mountainous areas like Austria and Switzerland. I use arnica to treat bruises and the effects of any trips or falls where the skin is unbroken. Marigold, St John's wort and camomile are more effective on open wounds and abrasions. A bath or massage with arnica oil is a wonderful way to ease muscle pain.

## Effect on the skin
Analgesic, diuretic (so it reduces swelling) and anti-inflammatory.

## When to use
For bruises, swelling, bumps and muscle pain.

## Active ingredients
Essential oil, bitter substances (including helenalin), resin, flavonols glycosides, tannins, choline and silicon.

## Use
Dried and fresh flowers and root for a tincture or compress. You can apply undiluted tincture to your skin. For a compress, add 40 drops tincture to half a litre boiled, cooled water. Fresh flowers for an oil. You can use the oil as a base for ointments.

**CAUTION:**
Arnica may cause an allergic skin reaction; if this happens, stop using it immediately.

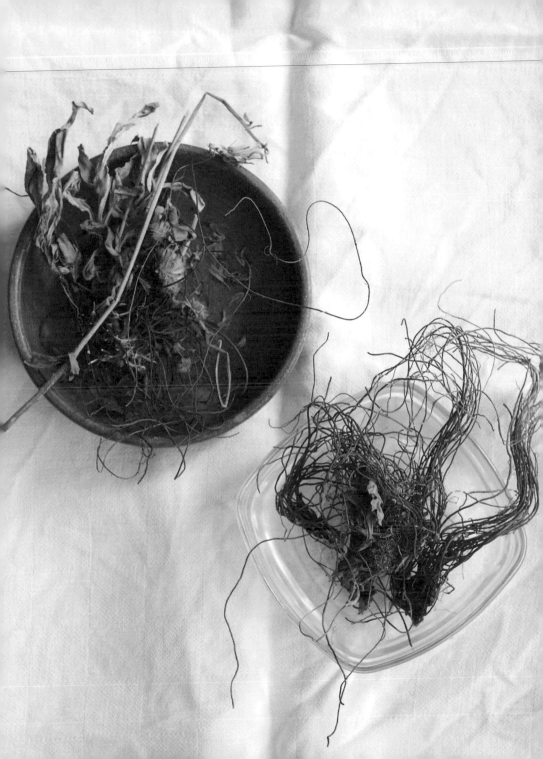

# MASSAGE OIL WITH ARNICA

# MAGNESIUM SPRAY

This oil is a wonderful way to enjoy a massage (self-administered or by someone else) if you are experiencing muscle pain.

Like arnica, magnesium also helps to ease muscle pain. You can apply the spray directly onto your skin.

**Ingredients for approximately 150ml**
- 50g arnica – dried flowers and root
- 100ml good base oil
- A clean 150ml pot or jar with lid

**Ingredients for 300ml**
- 10g magnesium chloride flakes or powder
- 250ml boiling water
- 50 drops arnica tincture
- A clean 300ml spray bottle

Place the plant parts in a dish, pour over the oil to cover them and leave in a water bath to infuse for 48 hours. Turn the heat off at night and on again the next morning, so you can monitor it consistently. Strain the oil, transfer it to the pot and it is ready for use.

The first step is to make the arnica tincture. Fill a clean pot with dried arnica root and plant parts, then pour over vodka to cover the material. Leave for 6 weeks with the lid on, shaking occasionally, then strain the tincture.

Pour the boiling water over the magnesium chloride and stir until it has dissolved. Leave to cool, then add the arnica tincture. Pour into the spray bottle and add a label.

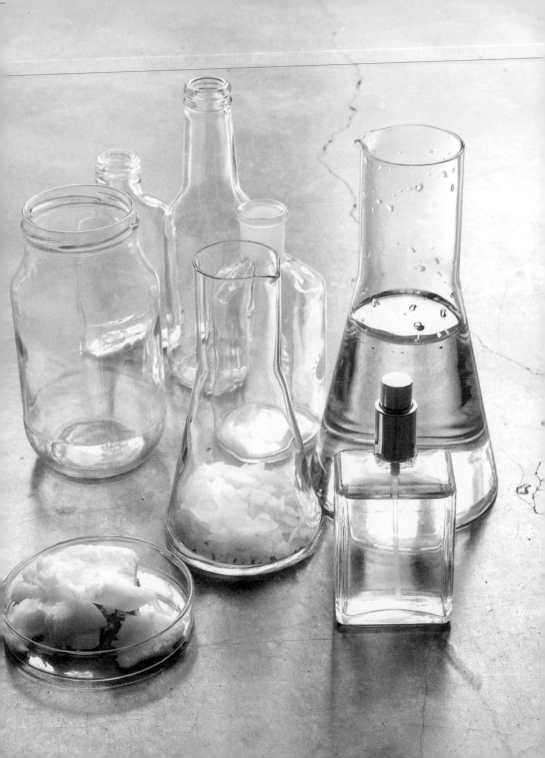

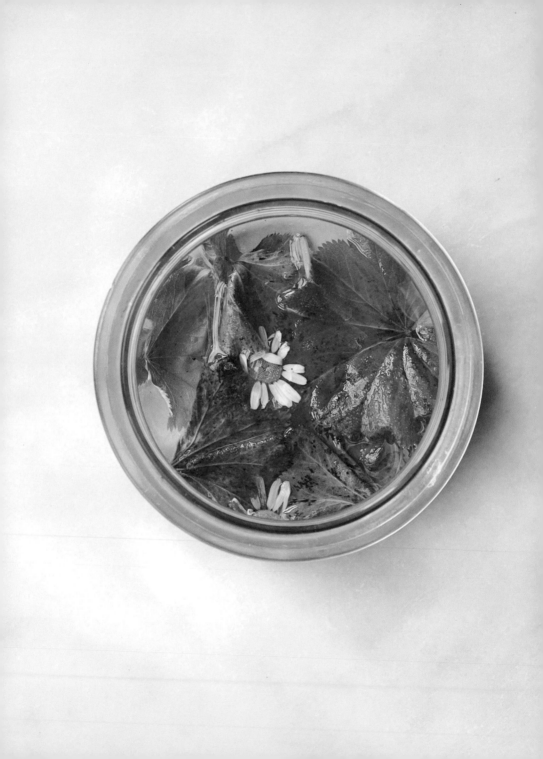

# OIL FOR YOUR INTIMATE AREA

You should only use gentle, natural oils with plants like camomile and lady's mantle on your intimate area; never use generic oils, essential oil or soap.

### Ingredients for 150ml

- 100ml organic almond oil
- Approx. 20g camomile
- Approx. 20g lady's mantle (enough to fill the pot when combined with the camomile)
- Two clean 150ml pots or jars, one with a lid

Fill one pot with the plant parts and pour over oil to cover them. Cover the pot with a cloth secured with an elastic band or a piece of string. Leave to stand for 4 weeks, stirring daily. Strain the oil, decant into the other clean pot, put the lid on and apply a label.

# LOOKING AFTER YOUR HANDS

## HAND CREAM

Treat your hands to a soothing cream that will nourish your skin and stop it drying out.

### Ingredients for approximately 150ml
- 50g beeswax
- 50g coconut oil
- 50g shea butter
- 10 drops vitamin E oil
- 10 drops essential oil, such as orange
- A clean 150ml pot or jar with lid

Place the beeswax in a water bath and heat until it is melted. Add the coconut oil and shea butter, allow to melt and mix thoroughly. Add the vitamin E oil and remove from the heat, then add the essential oil. Stir thoroughly and decant into the pot. Leave to set, put the lid on the pot and apply a label.

## HAND SOAK WITH FIELD HORSETAIL

Field horsetail (see page 129) nourishes and strengthens your nails, while camomile oil softens your cuticles.

### Ingredients for 1 bath
- 20g (one handful) field horsetail
- 150ml water
- 10 drops camomile oil

Bring the water to a simmer and cook the field horsetail for approximately 10 minutes. Add the camomile oil, then leave to cool slightly until the mixture is hand-hot. Immerse your hands for approximately 10 minutes.

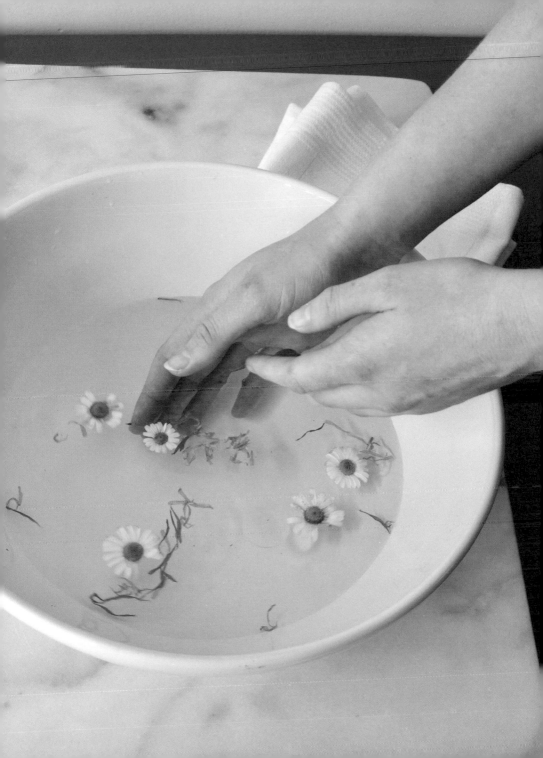

# LIZA WITTE'S HAND BALM

Liza Witte makes wonderfully fragranced skin oils and sprays to make your home smell delicious, as well as hand sprays and soaps. I discovered her products in a variety of shops, which all featured the unmistakable scent of her wonderful room spray. She likes to use fragrances that are associated with food and cooking, such as cardamom, chocolate and vanilla.

As well as having the magic touch with fragrance, Liza is also a stylist and potter (see opposite for pictures of her ceramics and page 223 for the ordering details). Whenever I visit her, her studio is filled with bottles and pots. She's been busy experimenting with little discs of hand balm that you can hold in your hands to nourish and soften your skin, inspired by the ones used by climbers to soothe painful hands abraded by gripping the rock.

Liza has generously shared her recipe for a rich balm for hands chapped by winter weather or the effects of working with soil and clay.

Liza: 'I call it hand balm for hard workers, climbers, potters and gardeners. This balm softens rough, chapped skin and can also protect your skin from the effects of heavy manual labour. When you hold the disc in your hand, your body heat melts it slightly. It's also really effective if you apply it before going to sleep, so it can sink into your skin overnight.'

## Equipment
- Precision scales
- Double boiler or a pan to heat ingredients in a water bath
- Two clean jam jars for melting your ingredients
- Two glass or wooden stirring rods
- Four small paper or silicone cups to use as moulds
- Four small tins for storing the balm

## Ingredients for four small hand-balm discs, each approximately 23g
- 33g beeswax, raw, yellow, in pieces and not deodorised (unless you don't like the smell of beeswax)
- 23g grape seed oil
- 22g sweet almond or apricot kernel oil
- 10g wheat germ oil (or 5g wheat germ oil + 5g sunflower oil)
- 3.5g cocoa butter

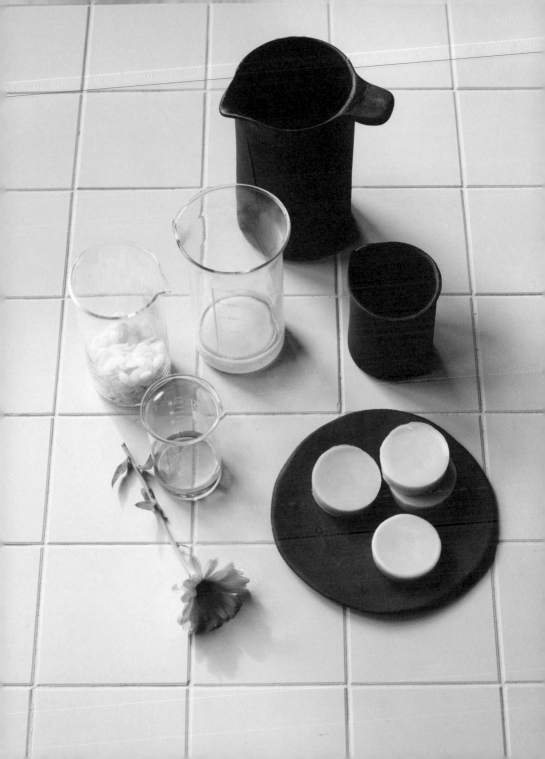

To get the best results, try to source cold-pressed and ideally organic oils. Most of the oils listed are available in health-food shops. Make sure that you weigh all your ingredients – including the liquids – in grams, not in millilitres. 100ml oil does not weigh100g! Be precise when you weigh the ingredients, otherwise the hand balm will be too hard or too soft.

## Required for extra fragrance

The discs themselves have a wonderful, gentle beeswax fragrance, but you can also choose to add 6–10 drops essential oil of your choice; I suggest frankincense, patchouli, camomile, myrrh, cedar and lavender. You can also make a maceration of your favourite plant with your favourite fragrance (see pages 12–13 for instructions). I suggest marigold, lavender, rosemary, vanilla bean or tonka bean (the tonka bean is the fruit of *Dipteryx odorata* and its fragrance is a blend of vanilla, almond, cinnamon and clove. You could use two or three tonka beans – whole, not sliced – along with half or a full vanilla pod in 50ml oil).

## Making the hand balm

Put the beeswax in a jam jar and heat in the water bath. Weigh out the other oils and pour into another jam jar. Once the beeswax is almost melted, place the jam jar with the oil mixture in the water bath as well and heat – but make sure it doesn't overheat. Once the beeswax is completely melted, pour the oil mixture into the beeswax and stir thoroughly. Add the essential oils (if using), stir again and pour the mixture into the moulds. Leave the discs of balm for approximately two days until they have hardened, then remove them from the moulds and store in the metal tins.

# HAND SANITIZER

This is the ideal way to disinfect your hands without using chemicals.

## Ingredients for 100ml
- 50ml witch hazel water (this is a decoction: see page 12 for instructions, and use the bark and leaves of the witch hazel)
- Approx. 25ml water (to top up the bottle)
- 10 drops St John's wort tincture
- 10 drops vitamin E oil
- 10 drops tea tree or lemon balm essential oil
- A clean 100ml spray bottle

Decant the witch hazel water into the bottle, then add the St John's wort tincture and vitamin E oil. Add the essential oil and top the bottle up with water. Shake thoroughly before using.

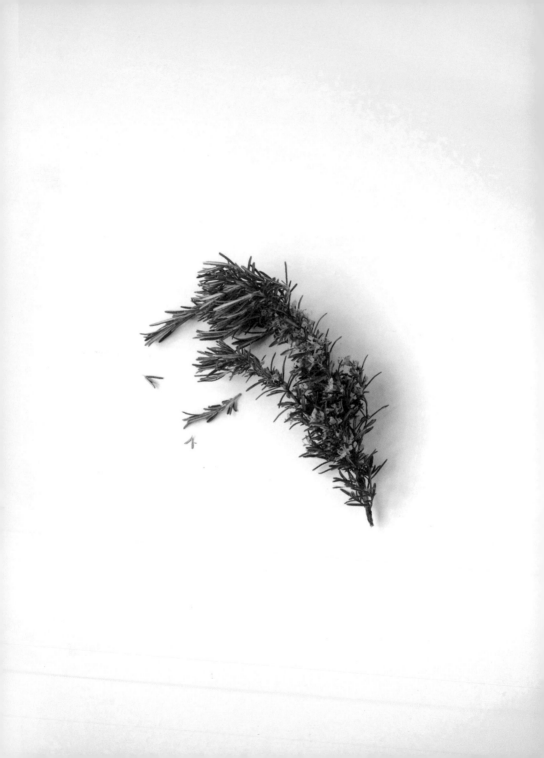

# ROSEMARY
## (Rosmarinus officinalis)

Lamiaceae

Rosemary is a sub-tropical bushy plant that also thrives
in Europe and has beautiful purple lipped flowers. The
energizing fragrance of the leaves stimulates your entire
system but also has a calming effect, so rosemary helps
you find balance.

## Effect on the skin
Improves circulation. The fragrance is both mentally
stimulating and soothing. Rosemary gets your nervous
system going, as well as your body as a whole.

## When to use
For chilblains and numb hands and feet, as well as for
tiredness, fatigue, low spirits or depression, mental
burnout and to aid recovery after illness.

## Active ingredients
Essential oils (including camphor, eucalyptol and
borneol), saponins, flavonoids, tannins, bitter
substances, calcium, B vitamins and rosmarinic acid.

## Use
Leaves and flowering tips.
Essential oil: the level of essential oil in rosemary
peaks just after flowering.
Harvest in August/September.

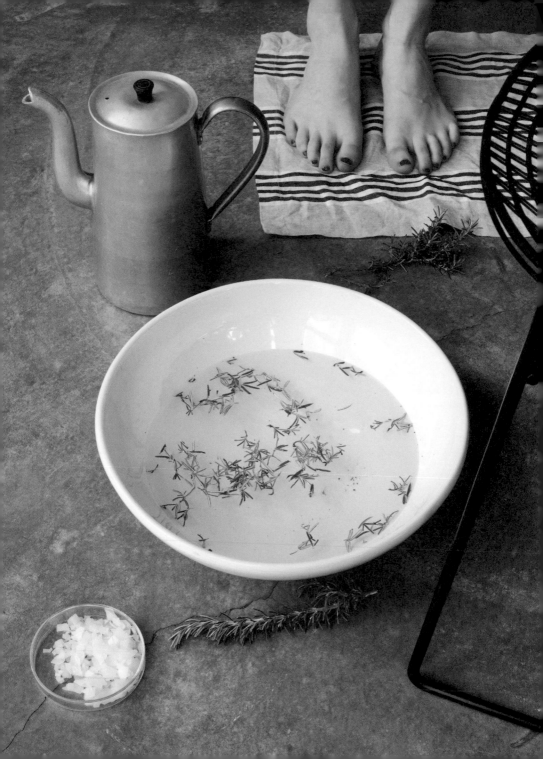

# LOOKING AFTER YOUR FEET

## FOOT BATH WITH ROSEMARY AND MAGNESIUM

Rosemary is very effective at boosting circulation so this foot bath is ideal for chilblains and numb hands and feet.

**Ingredients for 1 foot bath**
- 15g magnesium chloride flakes or powder
- 20g (1 stem) rosemary
- 500ml boiling water

Place the magnesium flakes and rosemary in a bowl and pour the water over them. Leave to stand for at least 10 minutes until the water has cooled to a pleasant temperature, then immerse your hands or feet for 15 minutes.

## FOOT BATH WITH HERBS

An excellent way to relax in the evening is to treat yourself to a foot bath - ideas for what to add to the water include:

- Calming camomile flowers or rose petals
- Antiseptic baking soda
- Calming essential lavender oil
- Antiperspirant essential sage oil
- Cooling apple cider vinegar

# FOOT OIL WITH MINT AND SAGE

This refreshing foot oil contains sage and mint to prevent excessive sweating and is effective against fungal infection. Apply after your morning shower or right before you go to bed.

### Ingredients for 50ml
- 50ml almond oil or another oil of your choice
- 10 drops mint oil
- 10 drops sage oil
- A clean 50ml bottle with cap

Pour the oils into the bottle and shake thoroughly to mix.

# FOOT POWDER WITH SAGE

A wonderfully cooling foot powder that prevents excessive sweating.

### Ingredients for 20g
- 10g (5 stems) sage leaves, dried
- 5g clay powder
- 5g cornflour
- Pestle and mortar
- Shaker

Grind the sage to a powder with the pestle and mortar. Add the clay powder and cornflour, mix thoroughly and pour into the shaker.

# OIL OR GEL FOR FUNGAL NAIL INFECTIONS

Treating fungal nail infections is tricky but this oil or gel is worth trying.

### Ingredients for 50ml
- 50ml almond oil (or another oil of your choice)
- For a gel, replace the almond oil with 50ml aloe vera gel
- 10 drops clove oil
- 10 drops essential rosemary oil
- 10 drops essential tea tree oil
- 5 drops essential eucalyptus or pine oil
- 5 drops essential thyme oil
- A clean 50ml bottle with cap

Mix all the ingredients thoroughly, pour into the bottle and apply twice daily to the affected nail.

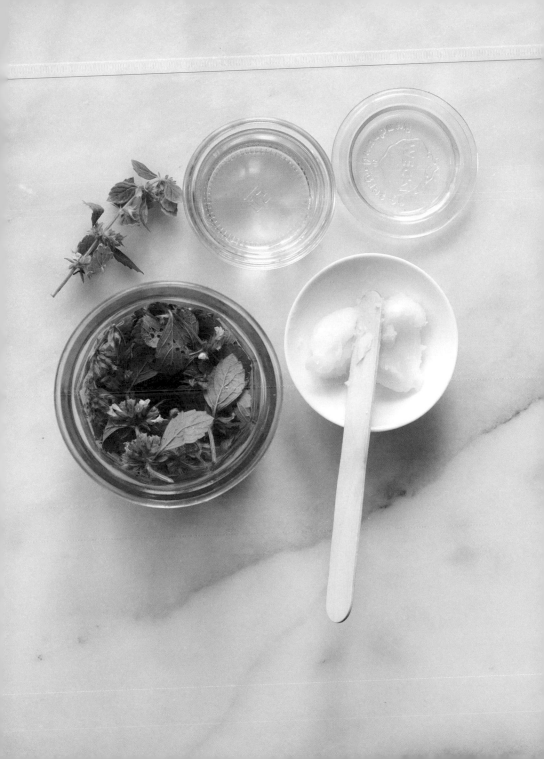

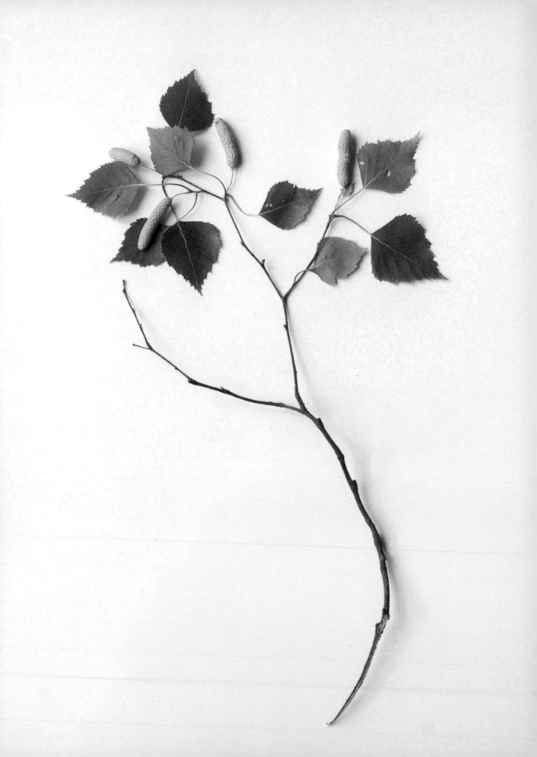

# BIRCH
(Betula)

Betulaceae

## Effect on the skin and hair
Cleansing and healing.

## When to use
For eczema, psoriasis, poorly healing wounds, erysipelas, venous ulcers and nappy rash, as well as for hair loss and dandruff.

## Active ingredients
Tannins, saponins, flavonol glycosides, essential oil, betulin, resin, minerals calcium and potassium, vitamin C, malic and citric acid.

## Use
The fresh, young, light green leaves in May and June.
Leaves and bark (including resin) for a tincture. The leaves for a tea.
The bark produces a resin that can be turned into an ointment or tincture.
Birch sap as a reinvigorating spring tonic. Only tap the sap in spring when it rises high in the tree; ideally when the moon is waning to stop excess sap loss from killing the tree. Always plug the hole afterwards with tree wax. The sap has a short shelf life.

# HEART'S EASE
(Viola tricolor)

Violaceae

## Effect on the skin
Soothing and anti-inflammatory.

## When to use
For chronic, flaking skin conditions like psoriasis, as well as for eczema (including in infants), cradle cap, nappy rash, oily skin, acne, blackheads, breakouts and itchy skin conditions. Can also be used internally.

## Active ingredients
Mucilage, flavonoids, anthocyanins, salicylic acid, phenolic acids, vitamins C, E and K, minerals and tannins.

## Use

The whole plant, harvested when flowering for a tincture or infusion. Make compresses and rinses.

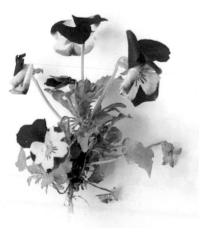

# COMMON COMFREY
(Symphytum officinale)

Boraginaceae

Common comfrey helps wounds to heal — even ones that are contaminated — and will speed up healing for broken bones.

## Effect on the skin
Anti-inflammatory and cleansing, encourages blood clotting, wound healing and tissue regeneration. Analgesic, prevents scarring, stimulates your circulation and counteracts swelling. Helps to prevent premature skin aging and helps maintain skin elasticity. Softening, soothing and hydrating for all skin types.

## When to use
For wounds, cracking, psoriasis, eczema, itching, contusions, bumps, fluid accumulation and haematomas. For acne, inflammation, sores, cracking and skin that is irritated, inflamed or damaged. Also helps with tendinitis, broken bones and muscle and nerve pain (including facial pain).

## Active ingredients in the root
Mucilage, allantoin, tannins, phenolic acids, phytosterols, pyrrolizidine alkaloids, amino acids, proteins, vitamins B1, B2, B3, B5, B12, C, D and E, minerals including calcium, potassium, phosphorus, iron, iodine, magnesium and manganese.

## Use
Fresh roots and leaves for a tincture. The entire plant, especially the root, contains pyrrolizidine alkaloids, which are damaging to your liver. The advice is to only use the plant externally and to avoid it if you are pregnant or breastfeeding. Leaves for an infusion or tea, or to rinse wounds. Grate the root and use to cover wounds.

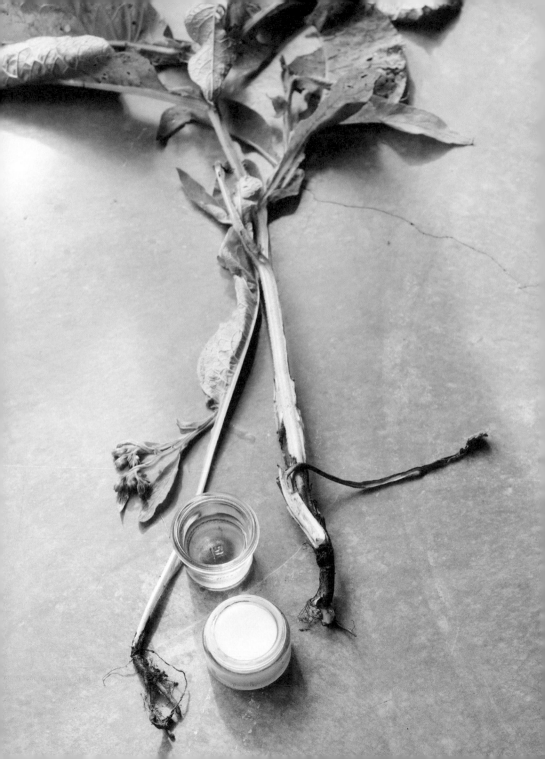

# COMMON COMFREY OINTMENT

You can use this ointment to treat the skin issues listed on page 201, as well as to combat skin aging.

**Ingredients for 200ml**
- 175ml coconut oil
- 100g common comfrey leaves and roots
- 15g beeswax
- A clean 200ml pot or jar with lid

In dry weather, pick the leaves of the common comfrey (dry them off if they are slightly damp). Dig up the roots, wash and dry them, then cut into rounds.

Heat the coconut oil and leave to melt. Add the leaves and roots and heat gently for one hour. Heat the beeswax in a water bath until it melts. Strain the oil and add to the beeswax, stirring thoroughly. Decant into the pot, wait until it has completely set, put the lid on and add a label.

# HORSERADISH AND HORSERADISH ROOT

## (Armoracia rusticana)

Brassicaceae

The root of the horseradish has healing properties and you can use it to draw splinters and inflammation from your skin.

## Effect on the skin

Boosts circulation and encourages skin to heal.

## When to use

For poorly healing wounds and raised scarring, as well as chilblains and numb hands and feet. As a compress for rheumatism, gout, nerve pain and muscle pain.

## Active ingredients

Essential oil, enzymes, flavonoids, coumarins, phenolic acids, vitamins B1, B2, B3, C, amino acids, carbohydrates and minerals including potassium, phosphorus, calcium, sulphur, silicic acid, zinc and iron.

# COMPRESS WITH HORSERADISH OR LINSEED

You can use either horseradish or linseed to draw splinters and dirt from minor wounds.

**Required for one compress with horseradish**
- ½ horseradish root
- Grater
- Compress

Grate the horseradish root and apply directly to the affected skin. Cover with a layer of gauze and leave overnight to penetrate.

**Required for one compress with linseed**
- 50g linseeds
- 100ml water

Pour the water into a dish, add the linseeds and leave for 20 minutes to soak. Apply the resulting paste to the wound or splinter, cover with a layer of gauze and leave overnight to penetrate.

## Use

The root, ideally fresh. You can eat both the root and the leaves.
Make a tincture as the base for a compress (dilute with water) or grate the root and apply it to your skin.

# FIGWORT
(Scrophularia nodosa)

Scrophulariaceae

Figwort grows everywhere but tends to go under the radar. Although large, it has inconspicuous flowers and an unpleasant smell. As you should not uproot or over-pick wild flowers in the UK, you will have to grow it yourself if you want to use it in your beauty products.

## Effect on the skin
Cleanses and encourages wound healing. Anti-inflammatory and reduces itching.

## When to use
For eczema, psoriasis and chronic skin diseases, as well as broken capillaries (including rosacea), varicose veins and piles.

## Active ingredients
Saponins, flavonoids, tannins, organic acids, glycosides, gum, resin and vitamin C.

## Use
The entire flowering plant (picked in the summer) and/or the root (harvested in the autumn) for a tincture. For a double tincture, start by using the flowering plant and then add the root in autumn.
The roots (thickest parts) for macerating in oil, which you can then use as a base for figwort ointment.

# OINTMENT WITH FIGWORT
# AND WITCH HAZEL

For better circulation if you suffer from broken capillaries, varicose veins or piles.

**Ingredients for 200ml**
- 100g figwort root (fresh or dried)
- 1 branch of witch hazel
- (or 100g bark and leaves, dried)
- 175ml oil of your choice
- 30g beeswax
- A clean 200ml pot or jar with lid

You can also replace the oil with coconut oil; if you do, you will only need 15g beeswax.

If you have figwort growing in your garden, dig up a few of the roots. Wash and dry them, then cut into rounds. You can also buy dried roots. Take a branch of witch hazel, remove the leaves and peel off the bark. Add this plant material to the oil, bring slowly to the boil and leave to simmer gently for 2 hours, then strain the oil. Melt the beeswax in a water bath and add the oil, mixing thoroughly. Decant into the pot and leave to set, then put the lid on the pot and add a label.

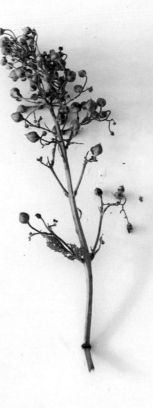

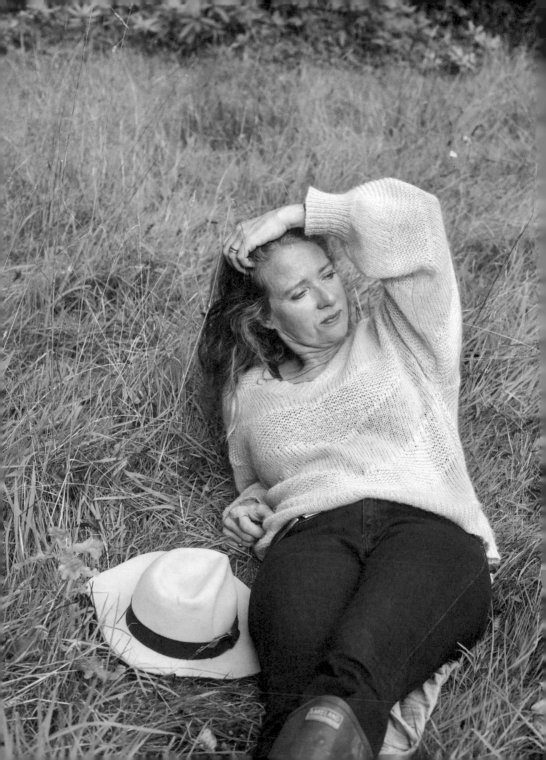

# BEAUTY COMES FROM WITHIN

Cleansing and caring for your skin is only half the story; you have to eat healthily as well. Covering that topic would fill a book on its own, so I'll stick to giving you some tips specifically for looking after your skin.

- Drink plenty of water or herbal tea.

- Take vitamin C supplements as this vitamin boosts collagen formation. Your body produces less collagen after the age of 25, resulting in skin aging and loss of condition and elasticity.

- Eat enough healthy fats, such as extra-virgin olive oil, walnut oil, oily fish, linseed oil, avocados and nuts.

- Make sure your diet is rich in antioxidants, including vitamin A (carrots and sweet potatoes), vitamin E (avocados) and carotenoids (like the red pigment in tomatoes).

- Eat plenty of zinc; a trace element that nourishes your skin from the inside. Your body cannot make this element itself, so choose food that is rich in zinc, including sesame seeds and nuts.

- Eat silicon (in oatmeal or nettles) to nourish your skin from the inside.

- Choose foods containing probiotics – including kefir, kimchi and kombucha – to encourage healthy gut bacteria, as neglecting your gut microbiome can cause skin problems, including eczema, psoriasis, acne and dandruff.

- Eat B vitamins in the form of wholegrains, nuts, seeds, dairy, fish and eggs.

- Last but not least, try to spend lots of time outdoors, get plenty of exercise and avoid stress.

# PRODUCTS FOR YOUR HOME

## ENERGY CLEANSING

The curanderos (folk healers) in Central and South America
use plants and herbs to heal and cleanse the energy of both
body and home. They use twigs, for example, and brush them
along the body, or burn plants and swirl the smoke around
you. They commonly use white sage for this, as well as
palo santo, which is the wood of the guaiac tree (*Bulnesia
sarmientoi*), but plenty of other plants are also suitable.
I like using local plants like pine, wormwood, common tansy,
hop clover, sage, rosemary, eucalyptus and lavender. Although
using plants like this is not common in the West, I do
recommend that you give it a try; surrounding yourself and
filling your home with wonderful fragrances is a delight.

Fragrances can stimulate or sooth your nervous system,
as well as cleanse the energy of your body and home. Try
burning, smoking or hanging up plants and herbs, or you can
use essential oil and an oil burner. All plants containing
essential oil affect your nervous system; some oils — like
lavender and linden — are calming while others — including
rosemary, thyme and marjoram — have a stimulating effect.

## BEDROOM SPRAY WITH LAVENDER OR PINE

This easy spray is the perfect way to relax and enjoy a
refreshing night's sleep.

**Ingredients for 100ml**
- 50ml vodka (with 40% alcohol)
- 50ml spring water
- 20 drops essential lavender
  (or pine) oil
- A clean 100ml spray bottle

Pour the liquids into the
spray bottle and shake to
mix. The spray is ready for
use immediately.

# AGUA DE FLORIDA

Agua de Florida literally means 'water of the flowers'. Created in 1808 by Robert Murray, it is one of the first natural perfumes. Its fragrance banishes negative energy, refreshes the energy in your surroundings and cleanses the energy of spaces and auras. This is my recipe for Agua de Florida.

## Ingredients for 100ml
- 50ml vodka (with 40% alcohol)
- 50ml spring water
- The peel of one orange, one lemon, one mandarin (or grapefruit), all organic and thoroughly rinsed
- Five stems mint
- Four stems rosemary
- Four cinnamon sticks
- Three star anise
- Two tbsp lavender
- A clean 100ml bottle
- A clean 100ml spray bottle

Place the plant material and fruit peel in the bottle. Pour over the vodka and top up with the water. Leave to stand for 21 days, then strain the liquid and decant into the spray bottle.

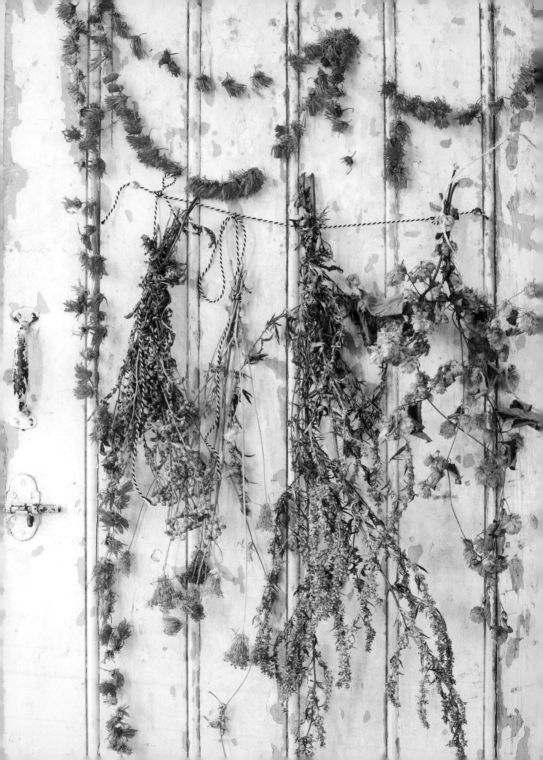

# PROTECTIVE HERBS

From smudge sticks (bundles of herbs that you light to produce smoke, much like incense sticks) that you use to cleanse the energy of your home to bundles of herbs that you use to protect your home or hang up to give it a wonderful fragrance, there are a thousand and one ways to create your ideal retreat. You could use cedarwood, for example, as well as lavender, wormwood, sage, common tansy and yellow sweet clover.

**Cedar** protects against unwelcome energies and stops moths from attacking your clothes.

**Common tansy** has protective properties and dispels unpleasant odours. It was used in the past to keep haylofts clear of lice and fleas.

Before carpets, **woodruff** was used as a floor covering so that the home would smell pleasant. It blooms in May and ushers in fresh energy.

**Jasmine** gives your home a wonderful fragrance.

**Yellow sweet clover** contains coumarins, which emit a delightful fragrance that calms your nervous system. White sweet clover is another plant that contains coumarins.

**Mugwort** protects against harmful energies. Its Latin name is *Artemisia vulgaris*, so using this plant in

your home is a nod to Artemis, the goddess of the moon and the hunt. She is also the goddess of nature and herb lore, as well as the patroness of pregnant women and women giving birth.

**Lavender** has a wonderfully calming fragrance that can also help ease headaches.

**Sage** is often used to cleanse and protect spaces.

**Rosemary** is stimulating and fortifying, and helps to drive out feelings of depression and melancholy.

**Pine and eucalyptus** are cleansing – including against bacteria and viruses.

**Hops** help you sleeps, so place a small bundle of them under your pillow at night.

# HERB SACHETS

You can make fragranced sachets to place under your pillow and help you sleep well – hops and lavender flowers are ideal.

**Ingredients for 2 sachets**
- 50g lavender or hop flowers (you can also add the essential oil from these plants)
- Sachets measuring approximately 5 x 5cm (sew them yourself)

Fill the sachets with the flowers, add a few drops of essential oil (if using) and then sew or tie up the sachet. Place it under your pillow when you go to bed.

# SMUDGE STICKS

Pick the herbs you want to use for your smudge stick; you can dry them, but you don't have to. Roll them into a cigar shape and wrap a cotton thread around it to hold it together. When you burn the smudge stick, place it in a metal or stone dish.

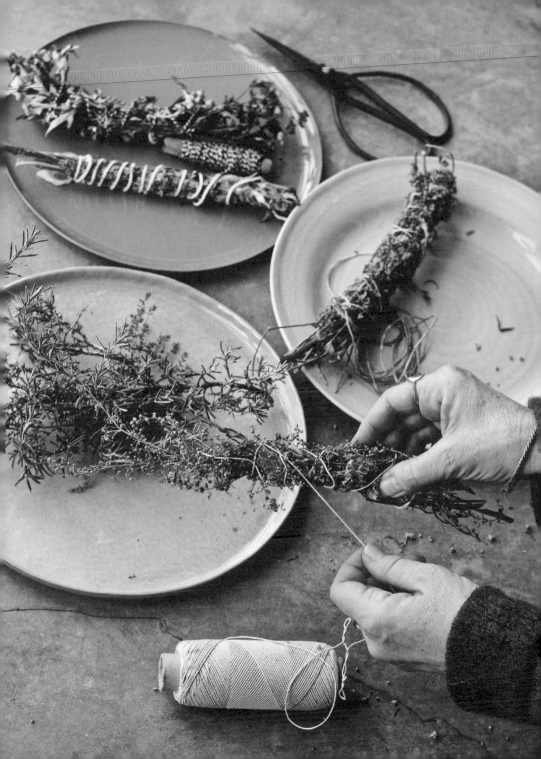

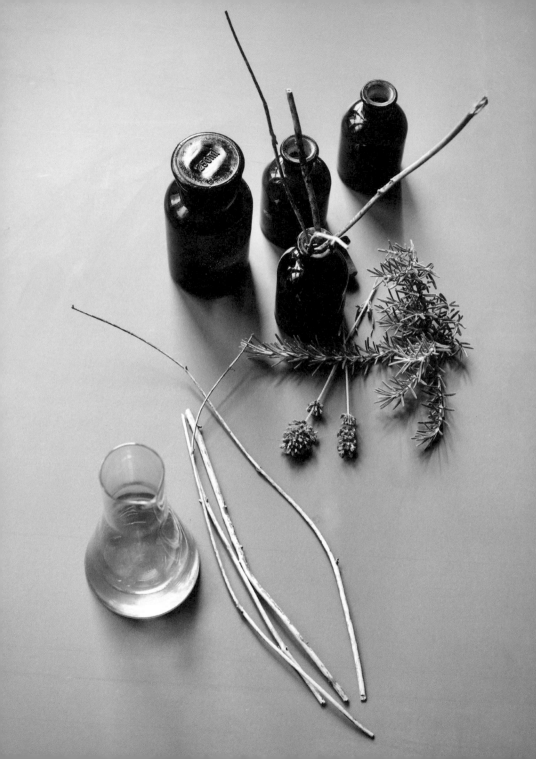

# NATASJA'S FRAGRANCE STICKS

Natasja van der Meer makes gorgeous natural products, from natural ink and pigments to fragrance sticks and sprays that you can use in your home. She also creates beautiful ceramics with natural glazes. Natasja had built up a following as a successful artist but her strong calling to only use natural materials led her to establish her business Native Nature.

Everything she makes looks absolutely wonderful; as if it was taken straight from the pages of a magazine. She has written a book about common nettles and has generously contributed her recipe for fragrance sticks.

Natasja: 'Although you can buy really great fragrance sticks, they tend to contain artificial fragrances and they are usually pretty expensive. Making your own fragrance sticks is quick and easy – and then you know for sure that they only contain natural and plant based ingredients.

'You can blend different essential oils to create your own unique fragrance, plus you can then choose a holder or vase for them that fits with your personal style. A glass or ceramic vase with a narrow neck will stop the fragrance from evaporating too quickly.

'Wooden skewers with the points removed are ideal for your fragrance sticks, but I really like using twigs that I collect during walks in the woods. Make sure that you remove the bark to make it easier for the fragrance to penetrate them. You often find twigs lying on the path where the bark has already come off; just keep a look out as you walk.

215

'The base for your fragrance is a vegetable oil that isn't strongly fragranced – like almond or sunflower oil. Mix the oil with alcohol; vodka, for example, which is odourless and has a high percentage of alcohol.

'If you want your vase to hold 100ml, mix 50ml oil with 50ml vodka. Add 50 drops essential oil of your choice, mix thoroughly and pour the fragranced liquid through a funnel into the vase. Insert between five and eight sticks or twigs and your fragrance sticks are ready!

# FRANK BLOEM'S FRAGRANCED CANDLES

Frank Bloem is a perfume maker and fragrance designer who operates under the name The Snifferoo, with creations including a sea air perfume for the Embassy of the North Sea and elephant fragrances for ARTIS Zoo in Amsterdam. He also gives fragrance and perfume workshops and readings about fragrances. He has shared his recipe for fragranced candles here.

Frank: 'According to the perfumery institutes in Grasse and Paris, being a skilled perfume maker does not necessarily make you a skilled maker of fragranced candles. Creating a good fragranced candle really is a skill in itself because fragrances behave completely differently in wax (including soy wax) than in alcohol. All of a sudden, the fundamental perfume maker's principle of top, middle and base notes no longer applies. Another factor is that the wax really subdues the fragrance, so you have to make a hugely exaggerated fragrance blend in order to create anything like a reasonable fragranced candle.

'I'm not talking about the fragranced candles you can pick up for 5 euros at IKEA or Blokker; most proper fragranced candles will cost more than 50 euros. That might seem ridiculously expensive to you, but if you look at how much perfume ingredients go into just one candle, that averages out at more than you get in a bottle of perfume. Put into context like that, then that price for a fragranced candle isn't so extreme after all.

'Fragranced candles are all about the melt pool; the bit of melted candle wax around the wick. The melt pool has to become as large as possible as this is where the fragrance is released. The flame incinerates the fragrance, so you can't smell it in the room. The softer the wax, the better it melts ... but the longer it takes to set again when the candle is snuffed. If a candle is too soft, it will sweat in warm summer weather. If your wax is too hard, you can soften it by adding some coconut oil. You have to pick the appropriate wick for the diameter of your holder and the wax you're using. If your wick is too thick, then your candle will smoke; if your wick is too thin, then the melt pool won't be big enough to release the fragrance.

'So there are plenty of factors to consider when it comes to making

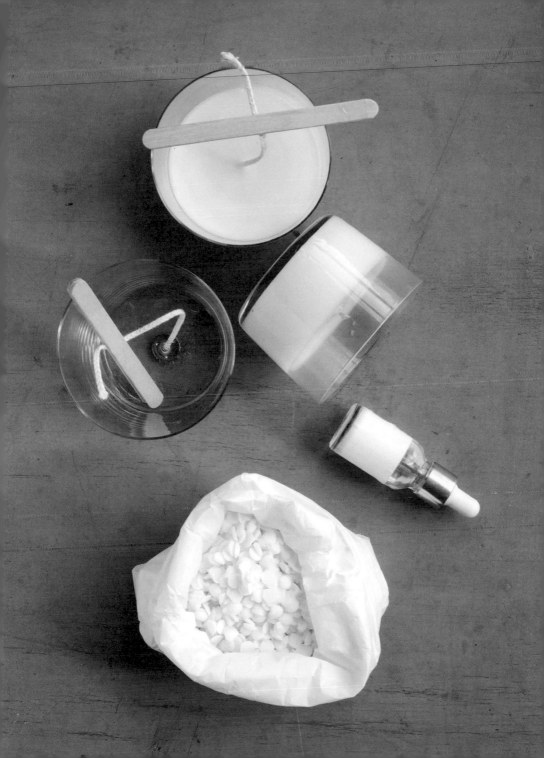

a good fragranced candle – and I haven't even got to the fragrance itself.

'A fragranced candle has two fragrances: the fragrance of the candle when it is lit and the fragrance of the candle when it is not lit. With an unlit candle, you mainly smell the fresher fragrance components; when it is lit, the heavier fragrance notes dominate. While the recipe I've shared only uses essential oils that you can buy in most health-food shops and chemists, you can choose from a wide range of natural and synthetic fragrances when you make candles.

'The ratio is 6% fragrance oil to 94% wax. You can increase the proportion of fragrance oil to 8% but using more than that is pointless; the wax cannot hold the excess fragrance and it will simply evaporate from the candle.'

### Recipe for the fragrance
• 40 drops essential lavender oil
• 40 drops essential patchouli oil
• 32 drops essential cedarwood oil
• 26 drops essential palmarosa oil
• 24 drops essential bergamot oil
• 20 drops essential juniper berry oil

The total quantity of drops of fragrance weighs 4.8g = 6%
That means the total quantity of candle wax is 75.2g = 94%. The candle as a whole then weighs 80g.

### Also required
• Soy wax* (organic, soft)
• Wick (with sustainer)
• Shot glass
• Heat-resistant pot
• Ice-lolly sticks
• Adhesive tape
• Measuring jug
• Weighing scales
• Spoon

*Soy wax is an alternative to beeswax and paraffin. It is made from soy beans; a crop that can be sown and harvested over and over again. As paraffin is made from petroleum, which is a fossil fuel, soy wax is more environmentally friendly because, unlike paraffin, no toxic substances are released into the air when it burns. Soy wax is a vegan alternative to beeswax. You can also use rapeseed wax.

Mix the fragranced essential oils in the shot glass, then melt the wax in a water bath. Use a dab of the melted wax to fix the wick sustainer to the centre of the bottom of the pot (or you can use glue).

Sandwich two ice-lolly sticks together and use adhesive tape to join them at one end. Thread the loose end of the wick between the sticks, rest the sticks across the top of the pot and carefully pull the end of the wick upward until the wick is stretched taut.

Place the measuring jug on the weighing scales and pour in 75.2g melted wax. Add the 4.8g fragranced essential oils and stir until the two are mixed thoroughly. Pour the fragranced wax into the pot and leave to set.

Potential issues include if the surface of the wax isn't smooth as it dries or – and this is more serious – if an air cavity forms just below the surface around the wick (so you can't see it). If you suspect an air cavity has formed, then use a wooden skewer to prick some holes around the wick. Direct hot air from a hairdryer onto the surface until the holes have filled with wax and the air has been removed. The candle will then look much more attractive as it dries. Once the wax has set, trim the wick to around half a centimetre above the surface of the wax.

Frank: 'This is all pretty straightforward. If you're a bit of a perfectionist, however, then making candles can become an almost never-ending quest for the perfect combination of wax, wick, pot and fragrance. The possibilities are definitely infinite when it comes to fragrance. Most people are satisfied with simply enjoying a creation that is not completely perfect and relaxing in the light of your gently smoking candle.'

Never leave a lighted candle unattended and always place it on a flat, level, horizontal surface. Watch out for pets, children, draughts and curtains blowing. When you light your candle for the first time, leave it to burn for a good long time so that the melt pool can get as large as possible.

# INDEX

221

## ACKNOWLEDGEMENTS

**Photo credits**
Anya van de Wetering: front and back cover, end papers, all interior photos with the exception of the ones listed below.
Bella Thewes: pp. 26, 27, 53, 67, 76, 80, 82, 97, 104, 105, 110, 126, 128, 130, 140, 179, 194, 198, 200, 201, 207

**With grateful thanks to**
Models Juna Krak: pp. 25, 175
Floor Janssen: pp. 39, 121, 142, 185, 190
Cathy Molenaar-Ursem, Angela Ursem, Food For Skin, foodforskin.care
Nele Odeur, Scent & Spice, scentandspice.nl
Frank Bloem, Snifferoo en.thesnifferoo.com
Marlies van Heusden, Nature bar, naturebar.nl/
Liza Witte, lizawitte.com
Michelle Dinger, The Ohm collection, theohmcollection.com
Jacqueline Sabaio, beekeeper

**Props for styling**
All glassware, cutlery, crockery, dishes and other items not specified are from the archive of Kamer 465 and Leoniek Bontje
Dille & Kamille, dille-kamille.nl: pp. 8, 12, 18, 37, 68, 70, 79, 93, 103, 127, 138, 145, 169, 176, 182, 190, 193
Plastic Free Amsterdam, plasticfreeamsterdam.com: pp. 54, 58, 113, 114
Rootfolk, rootfolk.com, handmade ceramics: pp. 123, 148, 149
Pastoe, pastoe.com: p. 190 Stadspaviljoen Noord, paviljoennoord.com: pp. 98, 99
Serax, serax.com: p. 54
Bensenhaver, bensenhaver.com: p. 38
Duikelman, duikelman.nl: p. 134
Edith van Gemmert: pp. 29, 98, 99
Van hier tot Tokio, japaneseantiquestore.com: p. 142
Helios, heliosholland.com: p. 214
Natural heroes, naturalheroes.nl: pp. 58, 114, 167

Ceramics by Warenhuis Vermeulen, warenhuisvermeulen.nl: p. 123
Ceramics by Liza Witte, lizawitte.com: p. 187 Soap and shampoo bars by Marlies van Heusden, naturebar.nl: pp. 123, 152
Candle wicks, wax soap moulds, online-zeepwinkel.nl: p. 217

**Locations**
Lady Lavendel, lady-lavendel.nl: pp. 24, 25
Koetshuis Waterland, koetshuiswaterland.com: pp. 2, 44, 45

**Basic ingredients**
Jacob Hooij, jacob-hooy.nl
Het Kruidenrijk, kruidenrijk.nl
Natural heroes, naturalheroes.nl
aroma-zone.com
arganolie.nl
online-zeepwinkel.nl
The Ohm Collection,
    info@theohmcollection.com
    (frankincense and myrrh)
lekkerhoning.nl

**Online sources**
https://kruiden.eang.eu/kruidenregister-
    fytotheek/zaailingen.com
www.palmolie.info/non-food/
https://tipsvoormama.nl/
mens-en-gezondheid.infonu.nl
plantaardigheden.nl

**Books**
Bontje, L., *Plant als medicijn* [*Plants as medicine*] (2021, 2nd edition, Terra, Amsterdam)
Bontje, L. & Noordermeer, Y., *Wildplukken* [*Foraging*] (2022, 3rd edition, Terra, Amsterdam)
Chown, V. & Walker, K., *The Handmade Apothecary* (2017, Kyle Books, London)
'*Healing remedies*', in *National Geographic*, March 2019

Kropf, I., *Het Kruidenboek van Ingrid* [*Ingrid's herb book*] (2016, 3rd edition, Grizzly Bear Guide, Eenrum)

Mabey, R., *Alle kruiden en hun toepassingen* (2007, 2de druk, Kosmos, Utrecht) / *The New Age Herbalist* (1988, Simon & Schuster Inc, New York, London, Toronto, Sydney, Tokyo, Singapore)

Maessen, Y., Kruiden - *signatuur en eigenschappen* [*Herbs – signature and characteristics*] (2019, 12th edition, Het Kruidenrijk, Haaren)

Uyldert, M., Lexicon der geneeskruiden [*Lexicon of medicinal herbs*] (1992, 17th edition, De Driehoek, Amsterdam)

Verhelst, Dr. G., *Groot handboek geneeskrachtige planten* [*Compendium of medicinal plants*] (2018, 8th edition, BVBA Mannavita, Belgium)

Gladstar, R., *Herbs for Natural Beauty* (1999, Storey Publishing, USA)

--